Pathophysiological Basis of Treatment in Convalescent Rehabilitation

Author: Masaharu Sato, MD.
Editor: Junji Taguchi, MD. Chief Director
Takarazuka Rehabilitation Hospital

文芸社

Pathophysiological basis of treatment in convalescent rehabilitation

Author: Masaharu Sato, MD.
Editor: Junji Taguchi, MD. Chief Director

Preface

In the acute care hospital, when the treatment of the main lesion is completed, if there is a limb movement disorder or cognitive dysfunction, the patient is early transferred to the convalescent rehabilitation bed. It is customary to send patients to convalescent rehabilitation hospitals without treating any accompanying pathologies other than the main lesion. As the length of hospitalization in acute care hospitals is rapidly shortened at present, it is unavoidable to allow time to address concomitant pathology. For this reason, although doctors in acute care hospital are experienced in treating the causative disease, they come to have little interest in pathological conditions other than the main lesion. Twenty percent of the patients admitted to our hospital in such a process are transferred to an acute care hospital again because of deterioration of their condition or other diseases discovered anew. It is often difficult to improve the patient's condition with the policy of performing only rehabilitation during convalescent rehabilitation, and more importantly, the underlying pathophysiology and risks must be well understood for rehabilitation doctor and also acute care hospital doctor, who will transfer the patients from acute care to rehabilitation hospital. I would appreciate it if the doctors involved comes to understand the underlying pathophysiology and risks. Otherwise, rehabilitation may be fundamentally inadequate, excessive for the patient, or it may be delayed to notice the progress or aggravation of the disease. One of the motives for writing this article is that young doctors majoring in rehabilitation and related fields can understand the above perspectives well and learn from this book to encourage their future studies.

Dementia, cerebral circulation disorders and infection are the most common in the convalescent rehabilitation territory as underlying diseases. In the first chapter of this book I have taken up cerebral circulation disturbance, which is the most common underlying disease in our hospital, and details its problems. Because I was able to acquire specialist's qualifications from many academic societies (Dementia Society, Stroke Society, Rehabilitation Society, Neurosurgery Society, Emergency Medicine Society (former)), I am proud that I am able to provide treatments from a wide range of standpoints, including both medical care for an acute phase and convalescent rehabilitation. So far, no academic book has been found that takes up various problems inherent in convalescent rehabilitation and other fields from a new perspective that connects the two fields. Most of the textbooks written by doctors who are said to be authoritative are not interesting to read because they only contain safe things. Perhaps I feel that those doctors are a little far from the front line of medicine in the ward. This book eliminates those shortcomings and presents my own, unbiased opinion based on my experience. In other words, I want to show you the new way of thinking and strategy of treatments. This is my second motivation for writing this article.

The reason why I decided to write in English is that when I entered department of neurosurgery, 80% of the superiors in the department had overseas study experience, so it was only natural even for me to learn about neurosurgery from academic textbooks in English, which might have depended on less Japanese textbook for Neurosurgery, and most of conferences seemed to be conducted in English. In such an atmosphere, I immersed myself in reading famous textbooks such as Diagnostic Neuroradiology by Taveras JM and Wood EH (1976), Radiology of the Skull and Brain by Newton TH and Potts DG (1972), and Microneurosurgery by Yasargil MG (1987), which every neurosurgeon knows. These medical textbooks differed from British and American literary books in that most of them consisted of a series of medical terms specially related to neurosurgery, which were relatively easy to read through. This reading experience gave me a lot of confidence not only for my neurosurgical specialist examination, but also for studying abroad in a foreign country when I was young. Today's young doctors are more familiar with English than we were, and the number of medical staff with overseas experience is gradually increasing around me. This is the third motivation for writing this article in English and that's why I highly recommend it. Incidentally, I should be grateful to Director Junji Taguchi, who studied abroad in the same institute after my studying abroad, gave me a great deal of advice on the completion of this book as an editor.

Finally, I would like to express my gratitude to Dr. Suguru Oomuro (the Chairman of Showakai Medical Corporation), Dr. Norimitsu Nasu (Honorary Director of Takarazuka Daiichi Hospital), Dr. Akira Nasu (Director of Takarazuka Daiichi Hospital and Board Chairman), hospital doctors, therapists, nurses, care staff, medical social workers, and other staff members of each department, who gladly gave me the opportunity to have this kind of clinical experience.

October 1, 2024 Masaharu Sato, M.D.

Eighty percent of the doctors, therapists, and nurses involved in rehabilitation work in convalescent rehabilitation. Although the acute phase is also important, the main focus of rehabilitation is the convalescent phase. As acute-phase medical care continues to develop, staff working in recovery-phase rehabilitation are required to have a high level of knowledge. We work day and night to collaborate not only with doctors but also with many staff from various professions working in recovery rehabilitation, share advanced knowledge, and ultimately help patients return to their homes and society. Many books have been published on rehabilitation, but this book has a really different perspective from previous books. So far, we have accumulated a lot of translational research from fundamental research to clinical practice as the author said. It is thought that this has a large influence. I would be happy, along with the author, if readers could sense this perspective.

October 1, 2024 Junji Taguchi, M.D., Chief Director

Dedicated to our wives.

Table of contents page

Chapter1 Cerebral circulation disturbance

Chapter 2 Dementia

Chapter 3 Clinical stroke

Chapter 4 Novel coronavirus infection

Chapter1 Cerebral circulation disturbance

Chapter 1 discusses cerebral circulation disorders, or cerebral ischemia, in detail. In addition to cerebral infarction caused by impaired cerebral circulation, hemorrhagic lesions may increase intracranial pressure and decrease cerebral perfusion pressure, leading to cerebral ischemia and neuronal cell death. Brain tumors and other conditions are often battles with neuronal cell death. These conditions are not completely cured of SIRS and CARS, and in convalescent rehabilitation wards there are many patients in unstable conditions. If blood pressure drops, the cerebral blood flow (CBF) autoregulation mechanism is disturbed and cerebral circulation disorder occurs, which may adversely affects prognosis. Since these phenomena are frequently observed, it is necessary to deeply understand the pathology of cerebral ischemia.

Neurophysiology

§1 Cerebral circulation
Na-K pump (at rest)

In a normal state, nerve cells generate electric potentials differently when they are at rest and when they are active. First, at rest, the cell membrane has Na channels (Na pumps) that are normally closed, but this is a pump that constantly pushes (pumping out) Na ions entering the cell out of the cell. K ion channels are always open. Since Na ions are pumped out, K ions flow into the cell to maintain electrical balance, and the concentration of K ions is higher than outside the cell. The concentration of Na in nerve cells is 15 mM, the concentration of K is 100 mM, and the concentration of Ca is 50-100 nM, and the extracellular concentration is 150 mM Na, 5 mM K, and 1-2 mM Ca. The resting membrane potential is about -70 mv (polarized and negative inside the cell). In order to maintain this potential difference, ion pumps of Na-K-ATPase and Ca-ATPase work by consuming 40% of the total ATP produced in the cell. Depolarization occurs for some reason, and the phenomenon in which the potential approaches zero from the resting potential is called depolarization.

Active cell membrane potential

When nerve activity occurs, that is, when an action potential is generated, the Na channel opens and Na ions flow into the cell, causing positive potential inside the cell, that is, depolarization, and when this potential exceeds a certain threshold (although it depends on the type of nerve cell, in general, if the resting potential becomes higher than the resting potential by 15 mV or more (becomes more positive), the current will flow through the nerve fiber (all-or-nothing rule). At this time, K ions flow out of the inside of the cell instead. This is depolarization. In other words, depolarization is a phenomenon in which polarized resting potential (-70mV) approaches (goes back) to zero level from the resting membrane potential for some reason or other is called depolarization.

Calcium ions

The calcium ion (abbreviated as Ca) concentration outside the cell is normally 1 to 2 mM, and the concentration inside the cell is much lower (1/1000 level) and shows 100 nM. Ca are originally stored in the endoplasmic reticulum and mitochondria (Mt) among intracellular organelles. During nerve cell activity, Ca channels are opened and a large amount of Ca flow into the cell, increasing the intracellular Ca concentration (instantaneously increasing up to 100-fold), causing transcription, activation of Ca-dependent enzymes, and protein synthesis. , neurotransmitter release, excitatory transmission, muscle contraction, endocrine secretion, and apoptosis. Transcription factors such as nuclear factor κB (NFκB) and nuclear factor of activated T-cells (NFAT) for intracellular signaling become highly concentrated and affect protein metabolism. Even if the Ca level rises, the Ca is normally quickly discharged out of the cell.

Glucose, O_2 metabolism

Nerve cells are fed with glucose and oxygen from the bloodstream. Glucose taken into the cell becomes acetyl-CoA through cytoplasmic glycolysis, and 38 ATP is synthesized from 1 mol glucose and 6 mol oxygen in the TCA cycle in Mt. This is aerobic glycolysis:

$$1 \text{ glucose} + 6\ O_2 + 38\ ADP + 38\ Pi \rightarrow 6\ CO_2 + 44\ H_2O$$

+ 38 ATP. That is, 38 molecules of ATP are produced from one molecule of glucose. Glucose is oxidized by oxygen in the TCA cycle in Mt or the Krebs cycle to produce energy, which is called aerobic glycolysis, and chemically combines adenosine diphosphate ADP with inorganic phosphorus to produce ATP. The brain cannot store glucose or O_2, so these O_2 and glucose must be constantly supplied by the blood flow in order to maintain brain metabolism. In contrast, cerebral infarction results in anaerobic glycolysis: 1 glucose + 2 ADT + Pi → 2 lactate + 2 ATP (this will be explained later).

Neurons are significantly more vulnerable to ischemia than cells in other organs. Neurons depend on the supply of glucose and oxygen as energy sources. By producing ATP through aerobic decomposition of glucose and oxygen, neuron functions are maintained and cell survival is maintained. However, since the brain has almost no reserves for these energy sources, disruption of their supply can lead to cellular dysfunction or necrosis depending on the degree.

Cerebral blood flow (CBF)

If the cerebral perfusion pressure (systolic pressure - intracranial pressure) is in the range of 60 to 150 mmHg, cerebral blood flow can be kept constant by expansion and contraction of cerebral blood vessels (Sato M, et al: Stroke 15:91, 1984). This phenomenon is called as "CBF autoregulation." CBF is best maintained when the hematocrit value is 33%. In addition, in hypothermic anesthesia, hypothermia at 33℃ for brain protection is said to be the most suitable, and it has the fewest side effects. As an aside, astrocytes are stronger than nerve cells against ischemia. This is because astrocytes are superior in the accumulation of glycogen, the expression of antioxidant enzyme, expression of apoptotic inhibition factor.

Ischemia

§2 Well, if a cerebral infarction occurs here (onset of cerebral infarction), simply put.

Half of the diseases in convalescent rehabilitation wards are cerebral strokes, and cerebral infarction accounts for the majority of cerebral strokes, so it is necessary to understand the vulnerability of nervous tissue to ischemia. As with cerebral infarction, it is important to keep in mind the fragility of nerve tissue for myelopathy, disuse syndrome, femoral and vertebral fractures, and dementia.

For example, when the whole CBF stops completely, the electroencephalogram(EEG) is flattened out in 10 seconds (consciousness disappears within several seconds and generalized convulsions occur), the electrical activity of EEG waves stops within 20 seconds, and the cell membrane depolarizes in 1 minute (Fig.1,2). The normal ion balance is disrupted, intracellular ATP is depleted in 2 to 5 minutes, and ischemic changes appear histologically within 15 to 30 minutes. However, in the case of ischemia, global cerebral ischemia does not always occur, and clinically, there are many cases of cerebral infarction in a unilateral, localized area. Experimental studies have been conducted for middle cerebral artery occlusion. However, in contrast to small animals, whose grey matter account for 60~70% of the brain, large amount of white matter accounting for 50% of the human brain, so the results of these experimental studies cannot be necessarily applied to humans.

The main phenomena caused by cerebral ischemia are ischemic depolarization, excitatory cell damage, oxidative stress, secondary microcirculatory disturbance, inflammatory response, apoptosis, recanalization injury and the like. Gray matter is strongly damaged by Ca and glutamate, and white matter is strongly oxidatively damaged by free radicals. Cerebral ischemia causes anaerobic metabolism, and various metabolic disorders and phenomena begin. The normal cerebral blood flow is 60-70ml/100g brain tissue/min. When cerebral ischemia occurs and CBF decreases to 40%, protein synthesis initiation factors are affected and protein synthesis in neurons is affected. Then, suppression of protein synthesis begins. Furthermore, when it becomes less than that, protein synthesis is completely suppressed. Suppression of mRNA production occurs at 25-35 ml/100 g brain/min. Not only the skeleton of cells, which are mostly composed of proteins, and organelles, but also the enzymes and genes that control intracellular signal transduction are damaged. If it is not completely damaged, it will be repaired, but the repair will take a considerable amount of time.

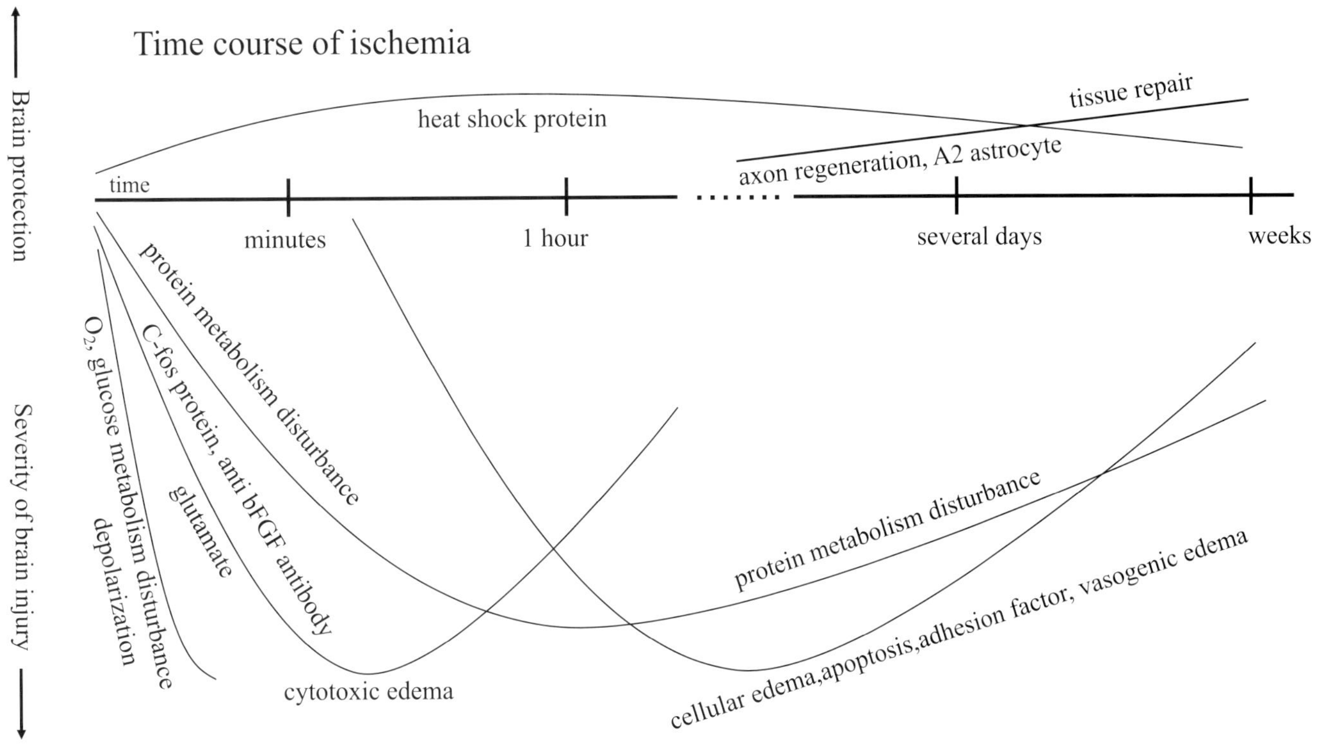

Fig.1.Time course of microcirculation during cerebral ischemia.

Cerebral ischemia leads to anaerobic glycolysis, which leads to ATP depletion, suppresses Na-K-ATPase, raises the cell membrane potential, and voltage-dependent Na channels open at once. Therefore, the intracellular and extracellular Na and K concentration gradients cannot be maintained. As a result, a large amount of Na flows into the cells from the outside, and depolarization becomes even more pronounced, leading to a decrease in intracellular K, lactic acid production, and tissue acidification. When CBF decreased down to 20ml, the resting membrane potential cannot be maintained (electrical failure). One to two minutes after ischemic depolarization, extracellular Ca enters the cell through voltage-sensitive channels. Electrical failure leads to ischemic depolarization of the membrane 2 minutes after blood flow is interrupted. When the CBF is further decreased to 10 ml, the nerve cell membrane is damaged (membrane failure), and the nerve cells become necrotic within about 5 minutes.

When cerebral ischemia occurs, brain tissue is stimulated by the action of C-C motif chemokine 2 (CCL2: CCL2 is produced from the ischemic area) and its receptor, C-C chemokine receptor 2 (CCR2). BBB disruption causes macrophage infiltration within the infarcted tissue. Microglia and macrophages produce inflammatory cytokines, and this inflammation lasts for several days. DAMPs derived from necrotic tissue of cerebral infarction include HMGB1 and peroxiredoxin (PRX). HMGB-1 is released 2 to 4 hours after ischemia, increases the expression of matrix metalloproteinase (MMP) 9, promotes BBB disruption, and further exacerbates inflammation. PRX is an antioxidant protein that metabolizes hydrogen peroxide into water within cells and has a cytoprotective function. However, it exits the cell and activates pattern recognition receptors on microglia and macrophages, inducing the production of inflammatory cytokines. PRX activates toll-like receptors and induces the production of inflammatory cytokines such as IL-1β, IL-23, and TNF-α, worsening inflammation. However, from one week after the cerebral infarction, microglia and macrophages produce anti-inflammatory cytokines such as IL-10 and TGF-β, acting in a neuroprotective manner, and begin to reduce inflammation and contribute to nerve repair (Wattananit S, et al: J Neuroscience 36:4182,2016). Furthermore, scavenger receptors (MSR1 and MARCO) expressed on microglia and macrophages recognize DAMPs such as PRX and HMGB1 and eliminate them from cerebral infarction tissue. Macrophages also produce neurotrophic factors such as insulin-like growth factor (IGF-1). Microglia and macrophages have a variety of functions, including inflammatory, anti-inflammatory, inflammation conver-

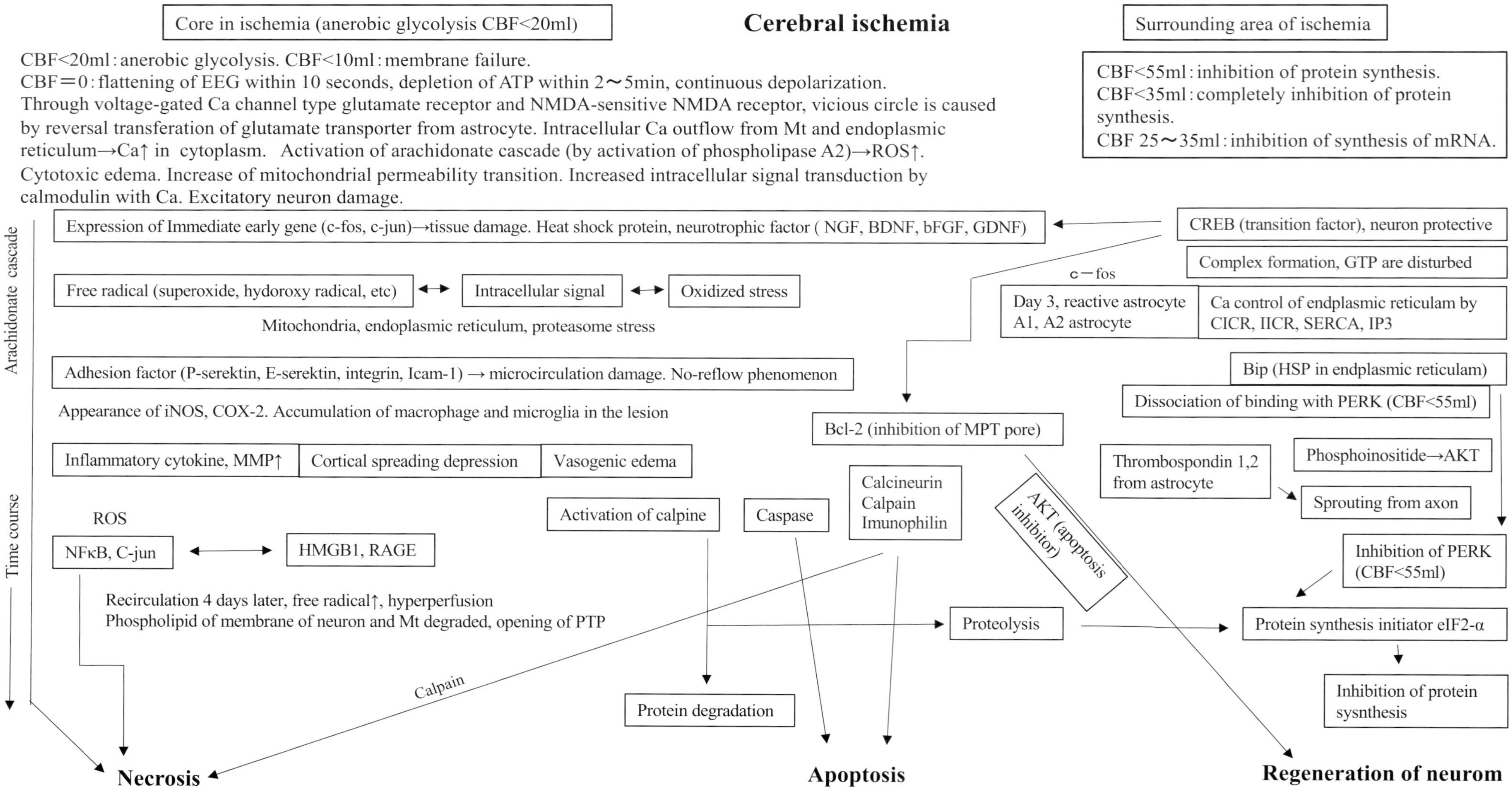

Fig.2.Microhemodynamics and intracellular signal transduction in cerebral ischemia.

gence, and repair, and play an important role in the progression of the disease depending on the stage of cerebral infarction.

When examined by MRI, intracellular osmotic pressure increased and intracellular edema occurs (low signal in ADC on MRI, high signal in DWI) immediately after cerebral infarction, followed by angioedema (high signal in both ADC and DWI) at 7 hours later. Incidentally, in the acute phase of epileptic seizures, MRI often shows high signal on DWI and FLAIR, and low signal on ADC.

Various genes are expressed in waves with cerebral ischemia, and are classified into four waves (stages). The first wave occurs in neurons in the early postischemic period. Among the immediate early genes, c-fos and c-jun are involved. The second wave is an expression group of heat shock protein-related genes, which occurs in both neurons and blood vessels, and acts as a cell protector. The third wave is the expression of inflammatory factor-associated genes, which stimulates the induction of adhesion factors with the expression of cytokines. The fourth wave is the expression of inducible nitric oxide synthese (iNOS) and inducible cyclooxygenase (COX-2). It plays an important role in causing nerve injury through ROS production. These reactions have a temporal width, are initially induced in the ischemic center, spread to the surrounding area over time, and are related to the phenomenon of infarct expansion. Cytokines arising by ischemia are RNF-α, IL-1β, IL-6, IL-8, MCP-9, CINC, IFN, p-selectin (cell adhesion factors), ICAM-1, ELAM-1, etc. Cytokines are produced from activated microglia and astrocyte.

Histologically, neurons are shrunken and scalloped within 30 minutes after ischemia, and swollen and vacuolated within hours. Along with this, neutrophils adhere to the vascular endothelium and invade the ischemic lesion. Macrophages appear within 2-3 days and show evidence of inflammation. Regarding ischemia, astrocytes are stronger than nerve cells. This is due to accumulation of glycogen by astrocytes, expression of antioxidant enzymes, and expression of apoptosis inhibitors. Spending more time till reperfusion evokes more damage as compared with infarction without reperfusion.

§3 If reperfusion occurs during this course (in simple terms).

Since ischemia cannot be considered if reperfusion is ignored, reperfusion injury is discussed in parallel with the discussion of ischemia. The primary treatment for ischemia is thrombus retrieval, which is exactly what is artificially causing reperfusion injury. While considering the adverse effects of this, we will consider the phenomena that occur with reperfusion.

If reperfusion occurs, the severer the degree of ischemia, the more irreversible changes tend to occur within a short period of time. While reversible, revascularization can rescue brain cells exposed to hypoperfusion. However, the therapeutic time window varies depending on the animal species and the experimental method. In general, the maximum of reperfusion initiation time is 1.5 to 2 hours after onset in order to minimize the damage caused by focal cerebral ischemia. In any case, restoring blood circulation as quickly as possible is the only means of minimizing brain tissue function and tissue damage. CBF of 10–12 ml/100 gm/min is typical numerical value for the degree of ischemia at which brain tissue can retain reversibility. Otherwise, it causes elevation of amino acids, membrane depolarization, lipid peroxidation, generation of ROS, elevation of intracellular Ca concentration, and various cytotoxic mechanisms.

Hyperperfusion occurs due to decreased brain autoregulation after reperfusion (Heiss WD, et al: J Cereb Blood Flow Metab 17:388, 1997). If the ischemic time exceeds 60 minutes, hyperperfusion is observed, and the possibility of death increases due to larger infarct formation and cerebral edema. Preceding severe ischemia and accompanying hyperperfusion exacerbate brain injury after reperfusion.

There is a concept of a neurovascular unit (the components of cerebral vascular endothelial cells, astrocyte, oligodendroglia, and neuron work together), and factors such as free radicals matrix metalloproteinase (MMP) 9 and tissue plasminogen activator (t-PA) disrupt the function of the neurovascular unit. Collapse of neurovascular unit may evoke the bleeding. Conversely, edaravone suppresses elevated MMP9 to make the neurovascular unit stronger (suppresses bleeding complications). (N-Acetylasparagine acid is a neuron marker).

MMP9 degrades cell adhesion molecules, plays a role in neuroplasticity and allows the formation of new synaptic connections. It also degrades amyloid β, but conversely destroys the BBB when its concentration becomes excessive. In the first place, MMP is a matrix metalloproteinase that acts to degrade extracellular matrices such as collagen and proteins expressed on the cell surface and to process physiologically active substances. Metal ions such as Zn and Ca are conformed to the active center of the enzyme. There are more than 20 types of MMPs, which are proteases (proteolytic enzymes) that decompose proteins.

§4 Glutamate receptor

Glutamate (glutamic acid) is the most common conductive substance among those that play the role of synaptic excitatory transmitters between neurons under normal conditions. Information is transmitted by stimulation. In the first place, glutamine is commonly converted glutamate by acid hydrolysis. Now, this glutamic acid in the synaptic cleft is taken up by adjacent astrocytes, converted to glutamine, transported to nerve cells, converted to glutamic acid again in nerve cells, and taken up into synaptic vesicles. Astrocytes have this glutamate transporter to protect neurons from the neuronal cytotoxicity of excitatory amino acids (Glutamate released with action potentials stimulates receptors on the post-synaptic membrane of neurons. Information is transmitted, and extracellular glutamate is taken into astrocytes and converted to glutamine. In short, it is recycling of the transmitter). This can keep the glutamate concentration outside nerve cells at a low level and protect nerve cells. Nerve cells also have this function, but astrocytes are the main ones. Receptors (so-called glutamate receptors) for the uptake of glutamate into cells include the following.

1. Voltage-gated Ca channel type ionotropic receptor, which indwells ion channels in the molecules.

① NMDA-sensitive NMDA receptor (N methyl-D-aspartate)

Due to its high Ca permeability, overstimulation causes neuronal cell death. NMDA receptors are closely involved in neuronal injury (so-called "excitotoxicity") due to excessive action of excitatory amino acids, and neuronal death after cerebral ischemia is due to this mechanism.

② Insensitive non-NMDA receptor

Non-NMDA receptors with low Ca permeability also allow Ca influx through voltage-gated Ca channels upon depolarization, resulting in excitotoxicity. A relatively mild chronic increase in extracellular glutamate concentration causes Ca influx. It leads to the generation of xanthine oxidase and generation of ROS, which accumulates molecular damage caused by ROS and causes cell death. It underlies chronic neuronal cell death and is associated with neurodegenerative diseases.

③ AMPA receptor (α-amino-3- hydroxy-5-methyl-4-isoxazole-propionate)

AMPA receptors are responsible for normal glutamate-mediated excitatory synaptic transmission. Because of their high Ca-permeability, the amount of AMPA receptors is an indicator of neuronal fragility (a large influx of AMPA receptors into cells causes excitatory neuronal cell death).

④ Kainic acid receptor KA (kainate) type

2. Metabotropic receptor (G protein-coupled receptor)

There are three types, Groups I to III, and the mechanisms of signal transduction vary depending on the group.

However, in cerebral ischemia or hypoxia, Ca-dependent glutamate release from the presynaptic membrane due to depolarization is followed by reverse transport of glutamate transporters (moving glutamate in astrocytes out of the cell). Reverse transport has a stronger effect on astrocytes than on neurons, and damages neurons. At that time, the problem is that a large amount of Ca flows into the nerve cells. When ischemia occurs, astrocytes cannot process them completely, and reverse transport occurs, and glutamate and excess Ca are present in the interstices, causing nerve cell injury.

Not only glutamate but also cytoplasmic Ca concentration is significantly increased from normal 50-100 nM to 1 mM, and many cytotoxic cascades are triggered. That is, proteolysis by activation of calpain, which is a Ca dependent proteolytic enzyme, activation of arachidonic acid cascade by activation of phospholipase A2, lipid degradation, free radical production, and various metabolic disturbance caused by activation of constitutive nitric oxide (NO)-producing enzymes, suppression of mitochondrial function due to Ca accumulation in Mt (Ca accumulation does not suppress Mt function), DNA degradation due to endonuclease activation, fluctuation of intracellular phosphorylation due to Ca/calmodulin-dependent protein kinase activation and the like occur. In addition, endoplasmic reticulum stress caused by depletion of endoplasmic reticulum Ca stores also induces various cytotoxic mechanisms such as inhibition of protein synthesis and induction of apoptosis.

As described above, during ischemia, excitotoxicity due to glutamic acid and a large amount of Ca flowing into cells is conspicuous in gray matter. On the other hand, this cytotoxicity is almost absent in white matter injury. This is because white matter lacks glutamatergic nerve endings (Shimada N, et al: J Neurochem 60:66, 1993). As I mentioned above in gray matter, glutamate and Ca are associated with cytotoxicity, and in white matter, axonal edema and oxidative damage due to Na ion influx are important.

§5 Calmodulin

Most of the proteins cannot bind to Ca by themselves, but can bind to Ca using calmodulin (which is also a type of protein). Calmodulin is expressed in the brain at a concentration of 10 to 100 μmol/l, binds to intracellularly elevated Ca, acts as a Ca buffer, binds to various calmodulins, binds to proteins and shows physiological functions. It can bind ubiquitous Ca and regulate many kinds of proteins, thus affecting various cellular functions.

One of the most important pathways is the activation of Ca/calmodulin-dependent protein kinase II (CaMKII) triggered by increased intracellular Ca. Ca-calmodulin-dependent protein kinases are serine/threonine protein kinases that are activated when the intracellular Ca concentration increases. CaMKII is abundant in nerve cells. CaMKII regulates the functions of proteins by phosphorylating neurotransmitter synthase, synaptic vesicle-associated protein, ion channel, neurotransmitter receptor, etc. and plays a role in changes in neuronal function.

Under normal conditions, the Ca concentration in the endoplasmic reticulum is determined by several ways. The first way is, Ca uptake from the cytoplasm into the endoplasmic reticulum by sarcoplasmic/endoplasmic reticulum Ca-ATPase (SERCA) while consuming ATP. The second way is through IP3 receptors which is on the endoplasmic reticulum cell membrane, and Ca is released into the cytoplasm (IICR) out of endoplasmic reticulum. The third way is ryanodine receptor-mediated Ca release from the endoplasmic reticulum into the cytoplasm (CICR). It is determined on the balance of 3 ways mentioned above.

During ischemia, this mechanism is involved and the Ca concentration in the endoplasmic reticulum drops sharply. As a result, incompletely processed proteins that do not fold normally accumulate in the endoplasmic reticulum. In addition, denatured proteins generated in the cytoplasm by the ischemic stress itself are also incorporated into the endoplasmic reticulum. As a result, malfolded proteins accumulate in the endoplasmic reticulum and bind to immunoglobulin heavy-chain binding protein (binding immunoglobulin protein, BiP), a molecular chaperone in the endoplasmic reticulum.

BiP, also known as glucose-regulated protein (Grp) 78, is a protein belonging to the heat shock protein (HSP) 70 group and abundantly present in the endoplasmic reticulum. After all, with the help of the chaperone called BiP in the endoplasmic reticulum, the protein is folded and processed appropriately, but the unfolded protein that failed to fold is refolded. Nevertheless, if it is failed to fold again, it is involved in endoplasmic reticulum stress, and regulated through PERK pathway, but probably it is led to oxidative stress finally. Among the molecules important for endoplasmic reticulum stress transduction, the phosphorylation of eukaryotic initiation factor (eIF) 2a through the PERK pathway via PERK molecules inhibits the formation of the protein synthesis initiation complex, resulting in inhibiting protein synthesis.

Increased intracellular Ca concentration plays an important role in ischemia-induced cytotoxicity. In addition, ryanodine receptor and inositol 1, 4, 5-trisphosphate (IP3) receptor on the membrane of endoplasmic reticulum was stimulated and it induces IP3-induced Ca release (IICR) and promote Ca release from the endoplasmic reticulum to the cytoplasm. In addition, intracellular ATP depletion suppresses Ca-ATPace on the endoplasmic reticulum membrane, and promotes Ca uptake into the endoplasmic reticulum. Furthermore, the increase in cytoplasmic Ca concentration activates Ca-induced Ca release (CICR), and releases Ca accumulated in the endoplasmic reticulum into the cytoplasm. As a result, Ca concentration in the cytoplasm is significantly elevated to 1 mM, triggering many cytotoxic cascades. High Ca concentration in the endoplasmic reticulum is required for various protein folding and processing functions.

§6 The glutamate Ca hypothesis

Excitatory amino acid (EAA) is a generic name for glutamate, aspartate, etc., and is an excitatory transmitter at synapses. It is a synaptic transmitter in most of the nerves. It is stored at the terminal portion of axon in the excitatory nerve covering the wide extent of the brain. Under normal conditions, the electrical stimulation that flows through the axon is received at the presynapse and EAA is released from the presynapse into the synaptic cleft, where it binds to the post-synaptic receptor. Glutamate that has flowed out into the synaptic cleft stimulates the post-synaptic membrane and is reuptaken by glutamate transporters which present on the surface of adjacent astrocytes to regulate its concentration.

However, during ischemia, glutamate is released due to the reversal action of the cell membrane glutamate transporter (the reversal action of the astrocyte glutamate transporter releases a large amount of glutamate into the intercellular spaces, causing damage to neurons). Increased extracellular glutamate concentration, which stimulates cell surface glutamate receptors, causes an influx of Ca as well as large amounts of glutamate into the cell. A large amount of Na also flows into the cell, resulting in further depolarization. That is, accumulation of extracellular glutamate causes intracellular Ca movement via NMDA and non-NMDA receptors as described above (within 1 to 2 minutes following ischemic depolarization). Many cytotoxic cascades are triggered by elevation of intracellular Ca. Many mechanisms of cell damage such as proteolysis due to activation of Ca-dependent proteases, free radical production, various metabolic abnormalities due to activation of NO-producing enzymes, mitochondrial dysfunction, DNA degradation, apoptosis induction, lipid peroxidation in or around cells, biological membrane damage, inflammatory reaction chain, adhesion factor induction, cerebral microcirculatory disorder, and protein synthesis disorder occur. Thus, ischemic neuronal injury such as neuronal cell death progresses further.

The process leading to the completion of such cerebral infarction is called cerebral ischemic cascade, and not only changes in various metabolic processes but also excitatory amino acids as described above are involved. These have already been mentioned. This hypothesis is called the glutamate calcium hypothesis, and is used to explain mechanism of the death of hippocampal pyramidal neurons after transient cerebral ischemia and the death of neurons in the penumbra area.

Glutamate released from astrocytes acts on glutamate receptor subtypes such as N-methyl-D-aspartate (NMDA) receptors, increasing the concentration of not only glutamate but also Ca in neurons, leading to cell death. Intraneuronal Ca rise causes activation of Ca-dependent proteases, calpains, which degrade cytoskeletal proteins. At the same time, calcineurin becomes activated, and through various mechanisms, the expression of fas-ligand (it especially occurs in activated T lymphocytes, but also in others) increases, causing neuronal cell death (a similar mechanism is related not only to pathological conditions of cerebral ischemia, but also to pathological conditions such as brain contusion and Alzheimer's disease).

During cerebral ischemia, ATP metabolites adenosine monophosphate (AMP), adenosine, inosine, hypoxanthine and other purine metabolites increase intracellularly and are released outside the cells. Adenosine rises when blood flow is reduced to 20 ml, but decreases rapidly after 20 minutes. Excitatory amino acids such as aspartic acid and glutamic acid increase when CBF is reduced to 20ml, but begins to be reduced after 15 hours. Adenosine controls the release of the excitatory amino acids outside the cells. It also inhibits the influx of Ca into cells (Matsumoto K, et.al: Brain Res 579: 309, 1992) (Matsumoto K, et al: J Cereb Blood Flow Metab 13:586, 1993).

In the evolution of ischemic infarcts excitatory amino acid accumulation such as prominent elevation of glutamate and exposure time has been considered an important factor for the infarct volume (Taguchi J, et al: J Cereb Blood Flow Metab 16:271, 1996) (Choi DW, et al: J Neurosci 7: 357, 1987).

Elevated extracellular glutamate levels that follow energy disturbances play a major role in cytotoxicity. This is explained by a theory called the glutamate calcium hypothesis. Various factors, such as shock proteins, expression of ROS, and changes in intracellular signaling, affect the course of subsequent cytotoxicity.

Glutamate release due to ischemia is decreased during hypothermia, and mild hypothermia is said to suppress ischemic neuronal cell death (see next session). Other than hypothermia, I can't think of a clear clinically useful answer for how to suppress glutamate-induced neuronal cell death.

§7 The arachidonic acid cascade

The astrocyte surrounds the synapse. Ischemia stimulates the metabotropic glutamate receptor on the cell membrane of this astrocyte, causing the increase of the intracellular Ca concentration and activation of intracellular phospholipase A2. From the phospholipid of the cell membrane, free fatty acid, particularly arachidonic acid, is released by this phospholipase. Consequently, the arachidonic acid cascade is activated and ROS production increased. As a result, various mediators are released from astrocytes into cerebral blood vessels, causing blood vessels to constrict or dilate.

Neuronal membranes are rich in polyunsaturated fatty acids that are susceptible to peroxidation, have abundant cerebral blood flow, and consume a large amount of oxygen, making them vulnerable to oxidative stress. In addition, Mt produce large amounts of free radicals, and Mt are prone to age-related damage. A large amount of iron accumulates in many sites such as the globus pallidum and the substantia nigra, and this tends to generate active oxygen. Antioxidant capacity is low because there are few antioxidant enzymes such as catalase in the brain. Astrocytes are connected to each other, but IP3, which increases Ca concentration through gap junctions, diffuses to adjacent astrocytes, causing Ca waves, which increases or decreases cerebral circulation. This Ca wave is related to cortical spreading depression (Tanaka K: Circulation Frontier 7:20, 2003).

An increase in intraneuronal Ca increases the production of large amounts of free radicals and ROS from the Mt, which in combination with the activation of caspases causes cell damage. Furthermore, increased intracellular ROS activates NFκB, and the release of inflammatory cytokines activates inflammation and immune responses. They exacerbate cerebral edema and microcirculation disorders. Cytokines produced by ischemia are produced from activated microglia and astrocytes, and are TNF-α, IL-1β, IL-8, MCP-9, CINC, and IFN. Adhesion factors are p-selectin, ICAM-1, and ELAM-1.

During mild hypothermia, the increase in free fatty acids, which is an index of cell membrane damage due to ischemia, was not suppressed, but the extracellular release of glutamic acid and free radicals were suppressed (Busto R, et al: Stroke 20:904, 1989) (Busto R, et al: Neurosci Lett 101:299, 1989).

§8 Penumbra and core

When a cerebral infarction occurs, there is a central core of necrotic nerve cells and a surrounding area (called a penumbra) that has not yet undergone a complete cerebral infarction. If the blood flow in the penumbra improves, function in the penumbra is restored (Astrup J, et al: Stroke 8: 51, 1977). This penumbra is an area showing an electoral failure but not a membrane failure. Glucose metabolism is completely impaired in the ischemic core due to the cessation of glucose and oxygen supply. Anaerobic metabolism causes a rapid increase in lactate and the disappearance of neuronal marker N-acetyl-aspartate (NAA), which can be revealed by magnetic resonance spectroscopy. On the other hand, in penumbra, although lactate appears due to anaerobic metabolism, the amount is low and NAA is retained. Diffusion-perfusion mismatch on MRI indicates an approximate penumbra between abnormal perfusion images and diffusion-weighted images (Fisher M, et al : Neurology 47: 884, 1996).

In order to reduce this area as much as possible, current thrombolytic therapy using thrombolytic agents (within 4.5 hours after onset), mechanical thrombectomy for endovascular surgery (thrombectomy is indicated within 8 hours after onset, but depending on the case even within 24 hours it is currently indicated and is carried out).

Misery perfusion (Baron IC, et al : Stroke 12:454, 1981) is a condition similar to penumbra when post ischemic state becomes chronic. There is a process of compensating metabolic disturbances due to decreased local cerebral blood flow (indicated by decreased oxygen metabolism rate CMR02 on PET) by increased cerebral blood volume and increased oxygen uptake rate. This area showing this process is a misery perfusion in a broad sense. However, when local cerebral blood flow further decreases in this misery perfusion, the increase in oxygen uptake rate reaches a plateau the compensatory mechanism exceeds the limit, the oxygen metabolic rate decreases down to the level at which the functions are disturbed. Ischemic penumbra is from this level with functional disturbance to the level at which cellular energy metabolism is impaired. Misery perfusion is present clinically, and is therapeutically useful concept.

In the chronic phase, the time span far exceeds the therapeutic time window, and ischemic penumbra is basically non-existent. In the stage infarction has only core with misery perfusion surrounding core. In fact, it is thought that there is an ischemic penumbra area surrounded by a narrow area of misery perfusion and changing to a core over time. Although there is a decrease in cerebral infarction, the rate of oxygen uptake is increased, the rate of oxygen metabolism is maintained, and nerve activity is maintained, that is, this area is essentially showing misery perfusion. This is outside the therapeutic time window in acute ischemic stroke. That is, in the acute phase, the penumbra occupies the area around the core. In the chronic phase, the penumbra does not actually exist, and most of its area becomes the core, surrounded by the misery perfusion area. In the area of misery perfusion, bypass surgery is performed to restore blood flow in the subacute to chronic phase treatment, which cannot be discarded (surgical indications are 73 years old or younger, Japanese EC/IC bypass study, JET study) (Kuroda S, et al: Stroke 32:2110, 2001).

The area of diffusion-perfusion mismatch in MRI is generally called a penumbra, but the area that can be rescued by reperfusion is thought to be larger than this area. The difference between penumbra and misery perfusion is; Misery perfusion in a broad sense increased OEF and maintained CMRO2. Penumbra is the area of OEF increase and CMRO2 decrease. However, it is sometimes called misery perfusion in a broad sense including both, that is, a region with increased OEF, and the area of penumbra is included in the area of misery perfusion in a broad sense.

Pathologically, the core remains necrotic and the symptoms of the core remain. Therefore, reperfusion as described above does not solve all problems; Neurological amelioration caused by core has naturally limitations. Since cell damage in the peri-infarct tissue persists for some time after reperfusion, it is necessary to treat further cell damage and protect the tissue even after the initial reperfusion period has passed. In practice, the time period during which various drug treatments are effective also depends on the individual circumstances. This time spans several days or more and is primarily supplemented by medical treatment. Therefore, in a broad sense, the therapeutic time window (a time period during which treatment is effective) is defined as a reperfusion window (a time period during which reperfusion is effective) and a cytoprotective window (a time period during which cell protection is required in the event of further invasive events).

For example, further cerebral infarction expansion may be seen early after the onset of cerebral infarction, and this is a phenomenon called spreading depolarization in which depolarization caused by penumbra of cerebral ischemia may spread to the cortex accompanied by decreased blood flow (Kumagai T, et al: J Cereb Blood Flow Metab 31:580, 2011).

In the penumbra area, various tissue injury mechanisms are induced after the onset of ischemia. First, oxidative disorders associated with free radical production, microcirculatory disorders due to secondary thrombus formation, infiltration of multinucleated leukocytes and macrophages, apoptosis which occurs in neurons and oligodendrocytes. Consequently, not only gray matter disorders but also white matter and myelin disorders are also involved.

§9 Signal transduction

How are signals from outside the cell, for example in stroke or in other diseases transducted? For example, in cerebral infarction or other diseases, extracellular signaling molecules (called first messengers) bind to cell surface receptors, and activate intracellular signaling pathways. Furthermore, it is transducted to second messengers (Ca, cyclic AMP, nucleotides, inositol trisphosphate (IP3), diacylglycerol (DAG), etc.), which play a role of intracellular signal transduction system, and transducted to target molecules in the cytoplasm and nucleus (signal transduction), exhibiting various effects.

Phosphorylation is a reaction in which a phosphate group is added to the hydroxyl group (-OH) of serine, threonine, and tyrosine residues among the amino acids that constitute proteins. It is called protein phosphorylation. Addition of a phosphate group often causes structural changes in proteins and plays an important role in controlling intracellular signal transduction.

Furthermore, the signals phosphorylate a part of intracellular protein molecules (serine, threonine, tyrosine, etc.). The protein exerts its function as an enzyme (it is called activation), and conducts stimulus to the next protein molecule, and repeats it. The protein molecules finally activate the transcription factor of the gene to express the target gene and express the function of the cell.

Signal transduction includes a variety of pathways, but generally begins with the binding of extracellular signal molecules to receptors on the cell membrane, followed by intracellular second messengers, and enzymes, delivering signal one after another. As the process progresses, the number of enzymes and molecules involved increases. Ultimately, it causes functional changes in cells, transcriptional regulation of specific genes by transcription factors in the nucleus, and cell death due to apoptosis. Such a chain of reactions is called a "cascade," and a small amount of input information induces a large reaction (functions specific to the cell, proliferation and differentiation of the cell, etc.). In addition, it may affect another path, and this is called "crosstalk." In some cases, it binds to receptors in the cytoplasm and directly regulates transcription.

In signal transduction, a signal is transmitted by phosphorylating a specific protein and changing its activity. That is, a protein kinase is an enzyme that adds a phosphate group (phosphorylates) to a protein molecule. Among kinases (phosphotransferases), kinases that phosphorylate proteins are called protein kinases. They are classified into tyrosine kinases, serine/threonine kinases, etc., depending on the position of phosphorylation.

That is, protein kinase is an enzyme that catalyzes the reaction of transferring the phosphate group of ATP to the hydroxyl group of serine, threonine or tyrosine of protein and phosphorylating the protein. Many enzymes in cells and proteins that perform various functions are activated or regulated by phosphorylation. These include protein kinase A which is activated by cyclic AMP as intracellular second message, protein kinase C, which is activated through inositol lipid turnover induced by Ca, and calmodulin-dependent protein kinase. Cells repeat reactions of phosphorylating and dephosphorylating intracellular proteins in order to maintain their functions. This phosphorylation causes the protein to change its enzymatic activity, intracellular localization, and state of assembly with other proteins. As described above, among amino acids, kinases mainly phosphorylate serine, threonine, and tyrosine residues. More than 99% of amino acids phosphorylated by kinases are serine and threonine (serine/threonine kinases). However, less than 0.1% of tyrosine phosphorylation (tyrosine kinase) is often more biologically important. The activity of kinases is finely regulated, and kinases themselves are subject to on-off regulation by phosphorylation. Dysfunction of kinases is often the cause of disease, and has been extensively studied, especially in cancer.

Now, I would like to digress a little from the main topic, but I would like to talk about upregulation. Up-regulation is a response to neurotransmitters, hormones, etc. by increasing the number of receptors or becoming hypersensitive to a decrease in stimulus caused by a decrease in a certain external substance or signal. Through the response mentioned above, up-regulation can be carried out. The process by which cells increase their ability to function and increase the amount of cellular components such as RNA and proteins. Conversely, down-regulation is the activation of a particular receptor by a molecule such as a hormone or neurotransmitter that reduces the expression of that receptor within the cell, making the cell less sensitive to that molecule.

§10 Intracellular signals

Let's see what factors exist in intracellular signal transduction and are involved in cerebral infarction. In addition to AKT and the transcription factor CREB (cyclic AMP response element binding protein, cAMP response factor binding protein), which act mainly neuroprotectively, there are signals such as c-jun and NFκB, which act and work cytotoxically. Upstream of this signal, intracellular Ca elevation, activation of second messengers such as cyclic AMP, and activation of various growth factor receptors are involved. Moreover, signal transduction is closely intertwined with free radicals. So which pathways of intracellular signaling are important for ischemia? Among the many signaling pathways, there are many related to ischemia, and all of them are important. However, it is impossible for clinicians to be familiar with all of them, so I took up the signaling factors that frequently appear when reading related books. Various signaling factors also appear in the following sections.

AKT, serine threonine kinase (protein kinase B)

In signaling pathways, AKT plays an important role in many cell survival pathways, primarily as an inhibitor of apoptosis, and also plays a regulatory role in angiogenesis and metabolism. In addition, it is involved in various cancers and is an area of interest for anticancer therapy, and has a significant impact on various diseases such as cancer, diabetes, and neurodegeneration.

CREB

CAMP response element binding protein (CREB) is a transcription factor (described below) that increases or decreases gene transcription. CREB is present in the nuclei or Mt of neurons and oligodendrocytes, and is one of the transcription factors that induce transcription into mRNA. Genes or proteins whose transcriptional activity is regulated by CREB include c-fos, which belongs to the immediate early gene, neurotrophic factors (brain derived neurotropic factor, BDNF), nerve growth factor (NGF), Mn-SOD that scavenges free radical superoxide, B-cell/CLL lymphoma 2 (Bcl-2) that is an anti-apoptotic factor, cytochrome c that is important for mitochondrial energy metabolism, and IL-6, etc. In Penumbra, CREB phosphorylation is enhanced in the nucleus of neurons, and the expression of the anti-apoptotic factor Bcl-2 protein and the neurotrophic factor BDNF are also observed in the cytoplasm. The proteins whose transcription is initiated by CREB phosphorylation tend to act to protect the brain during cerebral ischemia. (Tanaka K: Progress of Medicine 231: 352, 2009 in Japanese). CREB is also well known for its role in brain neuroplasticity and long-term memory formation, and has been suggested to be involved in AD.

What are transcription factors?

Transcription is the copying of DNA into mRNA by RNA polymerase (RNA synthetase). Transcription factors are a group of proteins that bind specifically to DNA, determine whether DNA is transcribed into RNA by an enzyme called RNA polymerase, and can activate or repress gene transcription. It activates (promotes) or suppresses the process of transcribing DNA genetic information into RNA.

Promotor

A promoter refers to the upstream region of a gene involved in the initiation of transcription (the step of synthesizing RNA from DNA). Basic transcription factors and RNA polymerase bind to the promoter region on DNA to initiate transcription. Administration of cilostazol, a phosphodiesterase type III inhibitor, enhances CREB phosphorylation in the substantia nigra and maintains dopamine and substance P in the striatum, thus preserving the swallowing reflex. That is, cilostazol has a CREB activation effect. CREB phosphorylation plays an important role in neural tissue development, differentiation, regeneration, repair, synaptic plasticity, and memory retention. When oligodendrocytes are subjected to ischemic stress, CREB phosphorylation is enhanced in the nucleus, and CREB phosphorylation is sustained in the penumbra region, resulting in the expression of the anti-apoptotic factor Bcl-2 protein. That is, CREB phosphorylation is important for the survival of oligodendrocytes in ischemia (the expression of oligodendrocyte progenitor cells is enhanced in this region).

NFκB (nuclear factor-κB)

Nuclear factor-κB (NFκB) is a transcription factor that plays a central role in the expression of many inflammation-related genes. Normally, it binds to IκB and exists in the cytoplasm, suppressing its action. When IκB is phosphorylated and dissociated by signals such as other cytokines, LPS, viruses, and increased levels of ROS, NFκB translocates to the nucleus and binds to the promoter regions of cytokines, chemokines, and cell adhesion factors to promote their transcription. On the other hand, IκB is degraded by the ubiquitin-proteasome pathway. That is, NFκB is activated by an increase in intracellular ROS level (change in redox state), which results in the expression of COX-2, iNOS, MMP, ICAM-1 and other inflammatory cytokines. That is, NFκB dissociated and reduced by IκB moves to the nucleus, promotes transcription, and suppresses apoptosis. NFκB is activated 24 hours after cerebral ischemia.

NFκB is activated by antigens, viruses, bacteria, inflammatory cytokines such as TNF, cerebral ischemia, stimuli that cause oxidative stress (H202, ultraviolet rays, radiation, glutathione deficiency, etc.), and binds to target genes, followed by expression of several phlogogenic material, cell adhesion factors, and viral genes. Thus, NFκB is an intracellular stress sensor (Mattson MP, et al : J Neurochem 74:443,2000). In most cells, NFκB binds to a protein called IκB, which inhibits translocation to the nucleus. IκB is ubiquitinated and degraded by the proteasome when its serine residue is phosphorylated.

NFκB has been implicated as an intracellular sensor for oxidative stress. Many reports have consistently shown that NFκB binding to DNA is increased in the ischemic brain. However, its role has been reported to be both damaging (Schneider A, et al: Nat med 5:554, 1999) and protective (Botchkina G, et al :Mol Med 5:372,1999) (Yu Z, et al : J Neurosci 19: 8856,1999), as described below. The activation of NFκB by H_20_2 was inhibited in catalase-overexpressing cells and conversely, was activated in Cu/Zn-SOD-overexpressing cells (Schmidt K, et al : Biol Chem 2:13,1995). Thus, it is interesting that the mechanism by which the intracellular redox state activates transcription factors differs considerably between NFκB and AP-1. NFκB itself is activated in the cytoplasm and translocates to the nucleus. On the other hand, in AP-1, expression of c-Fos/c-Jun in the nucleus and binding to DNA are indirectly regulated through MAPK activation and Ref-1, respectively.

NFκB is regulated by TNF and ROS. TNF activates NFκB by activating ikKs that phosphorylate IκB. Aspirin, non-steroidal anti-inflammatory drugs (NSAIDs)and IL-10 inhibit NFκB activation by inhibiting ikK (Schottelius A, et al: J Biol Chem 274: 31868,1999).

The reason why NFκB exerts various actions is that there are many target genes in its downstream. MnSOD, Bcl-2/bc-x1 and inhibitors of apoptosis proteins (IAPs) are known to have NFκB-binding sites in their promoter regions among proteins that act as cytoprotective. The following cytotoxic proteins have been reported to be at least partially regulated by NFκB: iNOS, IL-1, ICAM-1, CINC, IL-8, neutrophil adhesion promoter, COX-2, MMP9, heme oxygenase (He)-1, Bcl-xs (pro-apoptotic genes). That is, TNF/NFκB can act either destructively or protectively depending on the type of cells in which they are expressed and the conditions at that time. In general, they are thought to affect cytotoxic gene expression when expressed in neutrophils/endothelial cells/glial cells, and protective gene expression when expressed in neurons (Bruce A, et al: Nat Med 2: 788, 1996)(Mattson M, et al: Neurosci Biobehav Rev 21:193,1997)(Yu Z, et al: J Neurosci 19:8856,1999). S100 protein binds to receptor for advanced glycation endproducts (RAGE) and activates NFκB. Increased intracellular FR level activates NFκB, resulting in the expression of many inflammatory cytokines including iNOS and COX-2.

NFκB activation is anti-apoptotic in some cases, but destructive in cerebral ischemia. NFκB translocation to the nucleus by rat 4-VO (30 min)/reperfusion was observed in almost all neurons 24 hours later, but NFκB translocation to the nucleus was suppressed 72 hours later. NFκB activation likely leads to the expression of iNOS, COX-2, adhesion factors and other cytokines in the ischemic brain. The expression of the 45-kDa CD-95 ligand (Fas ligand) is up-regulated in a model of focal cerebral ischemia, and is thought to be one of the causes of apoptosis. The CD-95 ligand gene has an NFκB binding site. Therefore, it has been pointed out that NFκB activation may be involved in its upregulation (Vogt M, et al: FEBs Let 429: 67, 1998). NFκB activation has also been suggested to be involved in the upregulation of Bc1-x short, a pro-apoptotic factor (Dixon E, et al: Brain Res 776:222, 1997). Oxidative stress associated with reperfusion activates NFκβ, and at the same time, many mRNAs of various inflammatory cytokines that activate NFκβ are expressed. Such cytokines promote the expression of adhesion factors such as selectin and ICAM-1 in endothelial cells. The inflammatory cells which appear through the process creates a vicious cycle for the endothelial cells, because the inflammatory cells produces ROS and activates NFκβ and AP-2. However, NO suppresses NFκβ activation in each tissue upon reperfusion.

A representative transcription factor whose activity is regulated by redox control is NFκβ. NFκβ represses genes such as cytokines, adhesion factors, iNOS, COX-2 and Fas receptor.

§11 Free Radicals

Even inhaled oxygen, some of which is metabolized into molecules called ROS, can cause cell damage in excess. Therefore, various mechanisms (antioxidant action) are working to eliminate active oxygen in the body. Under normal conditions, ROS are quickly eliminated by antioxidant action, but if excess ROS that cannot be eliminated occurs, that is, "the state where the balance between the generation and elimination of active oxygen and active nitrogen (described later) is lost" occurs, this is called the oxidative stress. Excessive oxidative stress conditions oxidize and damage nucleic acids, proteins and lipids, impairing cellular structure and function. These ROS and reactive nitrogen species (RNS) are called free radicals. The causes of excessive generation of free radicals are unfavorable lifestyle habit such as irregular life, smoking, heavy alcohol intake, excessive stress, and unbalanced diet. In addition, exposure to stress due to external factors such as radiation, ultraviolet rays, metals, and toxic substances, internal factors such as hypoxia (cerebral ischemia) and inflammation are the cause of excessive generation of free radicals. In the future, they may cause obesity, lifestyle-related diseases, dementia, brain aging, cataracts, skin aging, arteriosclerosis, diabetes, PD, AD, bronchial asthma, cancer, etc.

Antioxidant enzymes are the first to tackle ROS scavenging. Antioxidant enzymes include superoxide dismutase (SOD), catalase, and glutathione peroxidase (GPx). If the amount of ROS generated in the body exceeds the amount that can be eliminated by this antioxidant enzyme, the next thing that confronts the ROS is antioxidant substances. Antioxidants include glutathione, bilirubin, and vitamins. When these antioxidants fail to eliminate ROS, ROS attack and damage DNA, proteins, and lipids. Molecules such as DNA, proteins, and lipids that make up cells are oxidized and denatured by ROS, impairing cell functions.

Hydroxyl radicals, which are highly reactive among active oxygen, are directly generated from water in the body when exposed to radiation. Also, as mentioned above, a part (several percent) of the oxygen that enters the body through respiration becomes superoxide, which is converted into oxygen and hydrogen peroxide by SOD and the like. Hydrogen peroxide is reduced to water by catalase and glutathione peroxidase. However, when hydrogen peroxide is not sufficiently eliminated, hydroxyl radicals are generated by the action of iron and copper. This reactivity is high and further, for example, oxidizes lipids to generate peroxyl radicals and increases lipid peroxides.

Nitric oxide (NO) is produced from the essential amino acid arginine by nitric oxide synthase (NOS), and exhibits physiological effects such as blood pressure regulation and signal transduction.

Among free radicals associated with ischemia, ROS which may cause oxidative stress includes superoxide $O_2 \cdot^-$, hydroxyl radical ・OH, peroxy radical ROO・, and hydroperoxy radical HOO・. Among free radicals associated with ischemia, RNS which may cause nitrosative stress includes nitric oxide NO・ and peroxynitrite $ONOO^-$.

Damage to biological components by active oxygen and active nitrogen causes base oxidation and chain scission for DNA, inactivation due to oxidation and nitration for proteins, and peroxidation for lipids.

Now, the relationship between free radicals in the brain is that white matter contains a large amount of myelin (70% of myelin is fat), so fat content is high at 55% (gray matter has a fat content of 30%), and lipid peroxidation occurs. Gray matter is highly susceptible to disability. In addition, since oligodendrocytes and myelin contain a large amount of iron, a large amount of free radicals are produced, lipid peroxidation is induced, myelin is destroyed, and axonal conduction is impaired.

The vascular wall in brain parenchyma is a site where many ROS are expressed, the blood-brain barrier is also destroyed, and the autoregulatory ability of cerebral circulation is impaired. White matter microcirculation is also susceptible to damage by free radicals. Superoxide, which is a typical free radical, is detoxified by the action of SOD, glutathione peroxidase, and catalase, but in the presence of metal ions, it transforms into hydroxy radical which is a more powerful free radical. The free radical NO has both protective and damaging effects on brain tissue. Superoxide has a higher affinity for NO than SOD and produces peroxynitrite, which exhibits a very strong oxidizing action and damages white matter myelin and axons. NO production not only in parenchymal cells but also in blood vessel walls increases after ischemia and reperfusion, and combined with peroxynitrite production. Hemorrhagic lesions appear after revascularization, and free radicals are thought to play a major role for the damage. Peroxynitrite disturbs the mitochondrial electron transport chain and causes activation of PARP. PARP is a repair enzyme for damaged DNA. However, since excessive activation of PARP requires ATP for DNA repair, it consumes NAD and energy, resulting in cell death.

Mt are the main source of ROS in the body, and Mt consume about 95% of the oxygen in the body, of which 1-3% is converted to ROS. Superoxide, which is one-electron reduction of oxygen molecules, is also produced by ROS-producing enzyme systems such as NADPH oxidase in phagocytic cells such as neutrophils and macrophages. Approximately 90% of superoxide which arises in the body is produced in the Mt.

Mt are the site of energy production in aerobic respiration, and ROS are constantly generated from Mt, which are eliminated by antioxidant enzymes to maintain redox (oxidoreduction) balance and homeostasis. Redox regulation is to protect the body from various oxidative stresses and maintain homeostasis by controlling the redox state of the body. Redox regulation refers to the regulation of enzymes, transcription factors, and signal information by changes in the redox state caused by oxidative stress. However, excessive generation of ROS and a decrease in antioxidant capacity due to ageing or disease can disrupt the redox balance and cause oxidative stress. Mt DNA is also considered to be vulnerable to ROS and is more susceptible to damage than nuclear DNA.

Antioxidant enzymes are as follows. SOD is an enzyme that disproportionates the superoxide anion O_2^- to oxygen (O_2) and hydrogen peroxide (H_2O_2), and have metal ions such as CU/ZnSOD and MnSOD in its active center. Cu/ZnSOD is normally constitutively expressed and abundant in all cytoplasms. Mn-SOD localizes to Mt and acts to protect cells.

Catalase (CAT) is an enzyme that dismutates hydrogen peroxide into water and oxygen ($2H_2O_2 \rightarrow 2H_2O + O_2$). Catalase activity is said to be high in the liver, kidney, and blood.

Glutathione peroxidase (GPX) is an enzyme that eliminates hydrogen peroxide and peroxides produced in the body in the presence of glutathione. Under physiological conditions, generated ROS are converted to H_20_2 by SOD and metabolized to H_20 and O_2 by GPX and CAT.

On the other hand, endogenous free radical scavengers such as vitamins C and E play an important role in removing excess active oxygen groups.

§12 Why is the brain susceptible to damage by free radical?

Why is the brain susceptible to damage by free radical? It is generally believed that brain/nerve tissues are more susceptible to damage by free radicals than other tissues. Halliwell & Gutteridge gave the following reasons for this in 1999 (Halliwell B, Gutteridge J: In:Free radicals in biology and medicine. Ⅲrd edition.Clarendon Press, Oxford,UK,1999).

1. A rapid increase in Ca is likely to occur during ischemia/energy deprivation due to the intense movement of ions through the cell membrane.
2. The release of excitatory amino acids and ROS production forms a vicious circle, and ROS inhibits glutamine synthetase in astrocytes and reduces extracellular glutamate uptake.
3. Due to high oxygen consumption in the brain, mitochondrial production of ROS is also high, and age-related damage to mitochondrial DNA (accumulation of mutations, etc.) is likely to occur.
4. O_2 is converted to O_2- with autoxidation of many neurotransmitters (dopamine, L-DOPA, noradrenalin, etc.). Iron is also contained in many proteins (cytochromes, ferritin, aconitases, tyrosine/tryptophan hydroxylase, cytochromes P450, etc.), and probably exists in certain brain regions (substantia nigra, caudate, putamen, globus pallidus) in large quantities in combination with ferritin. In brain injury, iron ions released from proteins due to decreased pH promote the Haber-Weiss reaction and lipid peroxidation.
5. Unlike plasma, cerebrospinal fluid does not contain proteins that bind free iron. After subarachnoid hemorrhage, oxyhemoglobin, which is released into the spinal

cavity by hemolysis of red blood cells in the hematoma, is involved in the development of cerebral vasoconstriction through two major actions: ROS generation and NO absorption (Asano T: In Cerebral arterial spasm, Wilkins RH ed. Williams and Willkins,Baltomore,190:1980)(Asano T, et al: J Neurosurg 84:792,1996)(Asano T, et al: Crit Rev Neurosurg 9:303,1999).

6. Nerve cell membranes contain a large amount of polyunsaturated fatty acids, so they are susceptible to peroxidation.

7. Monoamine oxidase localized in the mitochondrial outer membrane generates H_2O_2 and aldehyde through the following reaction: monoamine (RCH_2NH_2) + O_2 + $H_2O \rightarrow$ aldehyde (RCHO) + H_2O_2 + NH_3.

8. Brain tissue does not contain catalase, and its antioxidant capacity is not as high as other tissues.

9. Microglia, astrocytes, and infiltrating leukocytes secrete O_2-, H_2O_2, NO and cytokines.

10. The brain has several isoforms of cytochrome P450. Among them, CYP2E1, which is present in the hippocampus, substantia nigra, blood-brain barrier, etc., and decomposes organic substances such as ethanol, halothane, acetone, and carbon tetrachloride, is the most likely to generate ROS. CYP2E1 expression is enhanced by ethanol.

§13 Free radicals under cerebral ischemia

As intracellular Ca increases, unsaturated fatty acids (arachidonic acid, stearic acid, etc.) are released from membrane phospholipids, and O_2•-, H_2O, •OH increases by the release of neurotransmitter. In addition, O_2•-reacts with NO, which increases with the activation of the inducible nitric oxide synthase (iNOS) under cerebral ischemia, to form peroxynitrite, a free radical with strong histotoxicity. These induce peroxidation of membrane lipids, cerebral edema associated with cell membrane damage, oxidative modification of proteins, and DNA damage, resulting in neuronal necrosis and apoptosis.

Nitric oxide (NO) is a physiologically active substance and a vasodilator derived from the endothelium. It is produced by the catalytic action of nitrous oxide synthase (NOS) using L-arginine, oxygen and NPDPH as a substrate. NO, synthesized from L-arginine by NOS, is a vascular smooth muscle relaxant. It acts as a vasodilator and inhibiting platelet aggregation, inhibiting leukocyte adhesion, and improving microcirculation. NO activates guanylyl cyclase and promotes the production of cyclic GMP, which transmits information further downstream and induces various physiological effects. It also reacts with O_2- and exhibits cytotoxicity. In other words, it has both effects and side effects.

The synthase NOS has three isoenzymes:

1. neuronal NOS (neuronal type nitrous oxide synthase, related to synaptic plasticity),

2. vascular endothelial NOS (endothelial NOS, activated by hypoxia and shear stress. eNOS is constantly expressed. NO is producted in ischemia),

3. inducible NOS (iNOS is expressed in response to stimulation and generates large amount of NO. Under ischemia, iNOS reacts with superoxide to produce peroxynitrite (ONOO-), which is highly tissue-damaging). NO production derived from nNOS and iNOS has actions such as cerebral tissue damage, and expansion of cerebral infarction, while eNOS improves circulation and protects ischemic brain.

In the endothelial cell in penumbra, superoxide $O_2 \cdot^-$ is produced by NADPH oxidase of neutrophils activated by ischemia, and endothelial cells are damaged. In cerebral ischemia, free radicals are generated from the penumbra and slightly less from the core. The pericyte contracts and blood flow is interrupted (as a side note outside the endothelium is the pericyte).

In reperfusion

Free radicals occur during ischemia, but increases markedly with reperfusion. Ischemic neuronal injury induces the release of the excitatory amino acid glutamate and an increase in intracellular Ca, inducing the activation of calmodulin to produce ROS via nNOS. Also, activation of phospholipase A2 promotes the arachidonic acid cascade. During reperfusion, a large amount of blood is introduced into neurons that are in an ischemic ROS-producing state, and a large amount of oxygen is supplied, resulting in an explosive production of ROS, which damages Mt and cell membranes. Increased ROS production leads to impairment of intracellular signaling upon reperfusion.

§14 Stress caused by free radicals

Free radicals cause three types of oxidative stress: Mt stress, smooth endoplasmic reticulum (ER) stress, and proteasome stress, leading to cell death. In the case of cardiac origin, many free radicals are produced and this oxidative stress is very likely to occur. NO is generated from nerve cells, reacts with ROS to generate N_2O_2, produces various radicals, destroys the mitochondrial electron transport system, destroys the proteins and lipids of the Mt themselves, and eventually causes the permeability transition pore (PTP) opening. Then, it induces cytochrome C release, and apoptosis (cell death includes necrosis and apoptosis, both whose fates are controlled by Mt).

Radical scavengers, which have been developed as therapeutic agents (antioxidant) for acute ischemic stroke, are expected to reduce the severity of ischemic stroke due to their cerebral protective effects (antioxidant effects). A representative drug is edaravone, which prevents ischemic damage by removing free radicals and suppresses cell membrane damage.

By the way, rt-PA is a neuromodulator and MMP9 expression in the brain is induced. It has effects such as promotion of hippocampal long-term potentiation, upregulation of nNOS, activation of microglia, and activation of plasminogen. However, ischemic stress upregulates endogenous rt-PA and can damage the BBB. Edaravone reduces the adverse effects of rt-PA.

As a side note, a neurotransmitter is a chemical substance that is released to transmit a signal from nerve cell to nerve cell, and a neuromodulator is a chemical substance that is released to alter the effectiveness of this signal to be transmitted and control synthesis and release of neurotransmitter.

Hippocampal CA1 and CA3 regions are well-known for long-term potentiation, and by short-term, high-frequency electrical stimulation between the CA3 and CA1 synapses, the transcription factor CREB also acts, through the AMPA receptor and NMDA glutamate receptor. Synaptic transmission efficiency is increased and memory is improved. Long-term depression is the weakening or disappearance of transmission due to the continuous application of weak stimuli. Alzheimer's dementia can also be viewed as the accumulation of amyloid β in the hippocampus, which inhibits long-term enhancement of the hippocampus and causes cognitive decline (Rowan M, et al: Philos Trans R Soc Lond B Biol Sci: 358:821, 2003).

§15 Cell adhesion molecules

Cell adhesion molecules cause microcirculatory disturbance, no-reflow phenomenon, and thrombus formation during cerebral ischemia. Adhesion molecules are classified into several types according to their structural characteristics, and are overregulated during cerebral ischemia (up-regulation).

A typical example is called selectin, and generally selectin is expressed on the surface of vascular endothelial cells, and adjacent leucocytes adheres to the endothelial cells by the tethering, rolling and becoming sticky leucocytes. In particular, this adhesion factor is up-regulated in vascular endothelial cells.

Among them, E-selectin is expressed shortly after ischemia and persists even after reperfusion. Adhesion molecule expressed on vascular endothelial cells to which leukocytes adhere to the surface. A significant increase in E-selectin has been observed in infarction.

P-selectin is a glycoprotein expressed on platelets and vascular endothelial cells. It accumulates in α-granules of platelets. The P-selectin adheres to P-selectin glycoprotein ligand-1(PSGL-1) accumulated in Weibel-Palade bodies of vascular endothelial cells. P-selectin is upregulated by reperfusion after ischemia, and fibrinogen leaks out of blood vessels and reacts with tissues after reperfusion.

L-selectin is expressed in most leukocytes such as granulocytes, monocytes and lymphocytes.

Integrins are glycoproteins presenting on the surface of cells such as leukocytes and macrophages, and have a cell adhesion function that connects the intracellular cytoskeleton and extracellular matrix. It has functions such as cell spreading, blood coagulation, cancer metastasis, and tissue repair. Tissue-damaging iNOS is produced via IL-1β (an inflammatory cytokine). In this way, brain damage spreads due to cessation of blood flow and reperfusion in blood vessels. During cerebral ischemia, microcirculatory disturbance progresses through the expression of such cell adhesion molecules. Macrophages that have infiltrated into the brain parenchyma release inflammatory cytokines such as IL-1, IL-6 and TNF-α, causing brain damage. In addition, these infiltrating leukocytes release MMP and damage the extracellular matrix, exacerbating brain injury. MMP9 destroys the BBB. Within 24 hours by MMP2 (reversible), and after 24 hours by leukocyte infiltration and other factors, MMP9 is activated resulting in long-lasting breakdown. Rt-PA activates MMP9 to further disrupt the basal ganglia and induce hemorrhage.

Intercellular adhesion molecule 1 (ICAM-1) is an intercellular adhesion molecule that is always present at low concentrations in the cell membrane of leukocytes and vascular endothelial cells. It shows high value in subarachnoid hemorrhage and is considered to be related to cerebral vasospasm. Clinically, it is said that the risk of cerebro-vascular disturbance is high in patients with high concentrations in plasma.

§16 Necrosis and apoptosis

Cell death includes necrosis and apoptosis. In general, necrosis is passive cell death in pathological conditions, and apoptosis is physiological active cell death that occurs during development and differentiation. The morphological characteristics of necrosis are swelling of cell bodies and intracellular organelles, and extracellular release of cytoplasm due to disruption of the cell membrane.

On the other hand, in the case of apoptosis, disappearance and shrinkage/fragmentation of cell bodies (apoptotic bodies), aggregation of nucleus, shrinkage of cell, disappearance of microvilli on the cell surface are observed. They are phagocytosed by other cells, so extracellular release of cytoplasm does not occur. Apoptosis occurs not only in neurons but also in oligodendrocytes, and this is closely related to white matter and myelin disorders. Apoptosis takes several days to develop distinct morphological features. In some cases, only nerve cells die, and leaving glial cells unharmed.

Among signaling factors associated with necrosis and apoptosis, caspases are essential signaling substances (proteases) that induce apoptosis of cells.

B-cell/CLL lymphoma 2 (Bcl-2) is localized to the outer membrane of Mt and either inhibits or induces apoptosis, opening the MPT pore. There it plays an important role in promoting cell survival and inhibiting the action of apoptosis promoting proteins. It inhibits apoptosis by inhibiting the activation of caspases required for apoptosis. Both the dephosphorylation enzyme "calcineurin" and the protease "calpain" are Ca-dependently regulated and positioned at the initiation point of apoptotic signal transduction. In addition, calcineurin and immunophilin, molecules with completely different functional activities, are intricately intertwined and play an important role in the control of apoptosis and necrosis.

Regarding the mechanism of apoptosis in ischemia-reperfusion, disruption of homeostasis of Ca concentration is a trigger. Dysfunction of various intracellular organs (ER, Mt) occurs, and oxidative stress that causes DNA damage, changes in proapoptotic gene expression, and activation of protease such as endonuclease and caspase are involved to destroy the genome. In other words, oxidative stress (derived from ROS) due to reoxygenation after reperfusion and leakage (release) of cytochrome C from Mt to the cytoplasm occur, affecting the transduction system and enzyme reaction system (electron efflux from Mt which is released from apoptosis cells and ROS generation associated with cytochrome C release).

Regarding the relationship between infarct expansion and apoptosis after reperfusion, it is thought that when reperfusion occurs in the preceding ischemic region, apoptotic cells appear outside the infarct, leading to infarction.

Reperfusion stage or regeneration stage

§17 Mechanism of tissue repair after ischemia

After ischemia, histologically, the neuron becomes shrunken and shows scalloped fanning within 30 minutes, and furthermore, swollen swelling, and vacuolation within several hours. Neutrophils adhere to vascular endothelium and invade ischemic foci. Inflammatory findings such as the appearance of macrophages appear in 2 to 3 days.

Molecular biologically, immediately after ischemia, energy deficiency, glutamate release, etc. are produced, and several hours later, stress proteins, neurotrophic factors, apoptosis-related factors, etc. are produced. After 2 days, matrix protease-related factors are expressed, and after a few days, accumulation of neutrophils occurs, followed by accumulation of macrophages and microglia, and inflammatory cytokines and MMPs increase from these. Reperfusion effects appear during this time.

Specifically, the expression of immediate early genes (c-fos, c-jun, etc.) are seen immediately after ischemia, suggesting signs of repair of nerve cells and axons. Reactive astrocytes appears around the infarct on day 3 and reached a peak 7 days later. In addition, c-fos protein is expressed and the anti-bFGF antibody in these reactive astrocytes were positive (basic fibroblast growth factor (bFGF) is a cell growth factor that acts on cell differentiation and proliferation), indicating the existence of a repair mechanism (Taguchi J: Osaka University Knowledge Archive 377, 1991). In addition, neurotrophic factors are secreted from the pericyte to protect nerve cells.

The c-fos protein is one of transcription factors, exists in the nucleus, and functions to form and maintain the cell skeleton during cell development. It forms a heterodimer with jun and binds to activator protein 1 (AP-1) to regulate transcription. It is a gene that does not cause new protein synthesis but is generated by various stimuli transiently in every cell. Because various cascade reactions and phosphorylation occurs following the expression of c-fos, it is useful as a marker of neural activity.

Three to four days after that the mechanism in the direction of tissue repair begins to work (although immediate recovery from ischemia is not simple).

It has been assumed that peripheral nerve axons regenerate, but central nerve axons do not. That is, one of the factors is that the axon terminal of the central nerve forms a distorted mass called a dystrophic endball, that is, a glial scar, and that the mechanism of axon regeneration seen in the peripheral nerve is insufficient in the central nerve. It was proposed by the famous Cajal a century ago and was awarded the Nobel Prize in Physiology or Medicine.

However, it seems that this is not necessarily the case. It is true that the restoration is very poor. After cerebral infarction, there are three glia cells in the brain where the mechanism of tissue repair works: astrocyte (protection and transmission of nerve cells), oligodendrocyte (forms myelin sheath around nerve cell axons and plays an important role in jumping conduction), microglia (immune cells in the brain that control inflammation and immunity). When you have a stroke, there is a reaction to try to recover from the stroke. Among glia cells, astrocytes play an important role. Astrocytes become reactive in the peri-infarct area. The reactive astrocytes include A1 astrocytes (cytotoxic, secreting molecules that are toxic to nerve cells) and A2 astrocytes (neurotrophic, secreting molecules that have protective effects on nerve cells). The conversion from the former to the latter is associated with microglia activated by α-synuclein. That is, M1 (impaired type) and M2 (protective type) are secreted from microglia and act on A1 and A2, respectively (M1 induces damaged A1 astrocytes and causes neuronal cell death). Cytokines from microglia induce ATP-induced downregulation of astrocyte P2Y1 receptors and protective astrocytes are induced in the peri-infarct area of cerebral infarction. It was said that microglia and astrocytes aggregated in the chronic phase and created glia scars, inhibiting axonal growth, but this is not necessarily the case. Exosomes in the infarction act to regulate the ratio of A1 and A2, promoting functional recovery after cerebral infarction (Liddelow SA, et al: Nature 541: 481, 2017).

Apart from molecular biology, histologically, non-crossing conduction pathway compensation in the medulla of the corticospinal tract, formation of new pathways and synapses to nerve cells by axonal sprouting, temporary enlargement of the primary motor cortex by finger movement on the paralyzed side occurs with the task. However, both are more concerned with fine motor skills and have less to do with muscle strength. In clinical practice, there is also a phenomenon of blood flow diaschisis, and the involvement of the cerebellum in the process of improving paralysis has been suggested. In addition, there is a mechanism of interhemispheric inhibition (imbalance between left and right) in which motor recovery on the paralyzed side is delayed due to overactivity of the unaffected hemisphere, which is linked to CI therapy. However, in spite of the various studies that have been carried out, it is often not enough to reconstruct the lost neural circuits and restore their functions. Increased turnover of spines that receive synaptic input, elongation of axons (regeneration), sprouting of new axons from the middle of severed axons (sprouting),

sprouting of lateral branches from undamaged axons, etc. have been discussed, but not easily conclusion is reached. Research has shown these reorganizations in damaged corticospinal tracts. In addition, thrombospondins 1 and 2 released from astrocytes are said to be involved in axonal sprouting and synapse neoplasia after infarction (Liauw J, et al: J Cereb Blood Flow Metab 28:1772, 2008). In addition, cerebellar Purkinje cells contribute to improvement by regulating information transmission from the cerebral cortex.

In addition, compared to superficial fibers (superior longitudinal fascicle/arcuate fascicle, middle longitudinal fascicle, inferior fronto-occipital fascicle, inferior longitudinal fasciculus, funiculate fascicle, frontal oblique tract, fronto-striatal tract), deep-layer fibers (pyramidal tract, sensory tract, visual radiation, cingulate fascicle) have poor plasticity and are difficult to recover (Nakata M: Jap J Neurosurgery 31 supplement: 106, 2022, in Japanese).

Previous research on gait and balance control mechanisms in humans has revealed that the cerebral cortex, especially the supplementary motor cortex and its descending projection pathway, play an important role in bipedal locomotion and standing balance maintenance. Therefore, neurofeedback intervention targeting the supplementary motor cortex promotes recovery from gait and balance disorders after brain injury (Mihara M, et al: Neurology 96:e2587, 2021).

Briefly summarized, various phenomena occur at the molecular level of post-ischemia:

1) Appearance of immediate early genes, c-fos, c-jun, etc. are representative.

2) Expression of heat shock protein-related genes.

3) Inflammatory factors, related gene expression.

4) Expression of iNOS and COX-2 (involved in platelet aggregation, vasodilation, fever, regulation of vascular permeability, etc.).

§18 Regenerative medicine

Regenerative medicine after cerebral infarction is in the process of development, and part of it is being applied to clinical practice from translational research. Satisfactory opening of occluded blood vessels after cerebral ischemia does not necessarily lead to a favorable prognosis and often leads to futile or harmful recanalization (futile recanalization), which cannot necessarily lead to amelioration of cerebral infarction. It accounts for 20-67% (Horie N, et al: Jap J Neurosurgery 31 supplement: 105, 2022, in Japanese), and it is expected that regenerative medicine will become more active without relying on only recanalization. Regenerative medicine for residual ischemic foci is classified into the following three types.

1. Utilization of neural stem cells: Neural stem cells present in the periventricular, hippocampal CA1, and dentate gyrus are activated by ischemia, which is expected in the natural course, but may not improve outcome significantly.

2. Stem cell transplantation: Mesenchymal stem cells (They are obtained from iliac bone marrow, adipocytes, umbilical cord blood, etc.) are transplanted. The most common stem cell therapy is a bone marrow transplant; sometimes using umbilical cord blood. In the acute phase, Teijin and, Healios company, etc., and in the subacute phase, Sapporo Medical University, Tohoku University (intravenous administration of mesenchymal pluripotent stem cell 'MUSE cells'), Hiroshima University, Life Science Institute, etc. They are mostly done by intravenous administration.

Regarding mesenchymal stem cell transplantation at Sapporo Medical University, bone marrow fluid is collected from the patient's ilium within one month after the onset of cerebral infarction, cultured, and intravenously infused. This reduces FLAIR's high signal. When combined with rehabilitation, increased production of neurotrophic factors such as brain derived neurotrophic factor (BDNF) and increased receptors are observed. Most are single dose administration. Nerve regeneration is thought to occur shortly after treatment, or over several months or over a year (Sapporo Medical University).

In the subacute and chronic stages, intraparenchymal administration (stereotactic neurosurgery administration to penumbra and normal sites) is available (Hokkaido University; autologous bone marrow mesenchymal stem cell transplantation in the subacute stage). Transplanted cells migrate to the penumbra. In most cases, neuron protection is performed in anticipation of cytokine effects and inflammation suppression, and subsequent drug treatment is expected, aiming at a bystander effect as a bystander. Transplanted cells do not survive long term.

3. Stem cell transplantation using embryonic stem cell transplantation (human ES/iPS cells): That is, they isolate and culture embryonic stem cells (ES cells), generating stem cells using somatic cell nuclear transfer, and generating iPS cells in the development of stem cell therapy. Instead of helping necrotic cells, they create new corticospinal tracts, and transplant to a penumbra or new site instead of the core. Human ES cells are cultured for 6 to 10 weeks to create a layered structure or mini-organ (induction of cerebral organoids), then transplanted with a thicker layer to extend axons from the cerebrum to the spinal cord. Similar to 1 and 2 above, combined use of rehabilitation is effective (Kyoto University).

§19 Neurotrophic factors

Neurotrophic factors play essential roles in the normal development and differentiation of neurons and survival of mature cells. Neurotrophic factors are protein peptides and their receptors include tyrosine kinase receptors, cytokine receptors, serine/threonine kinase receptors and the like. Neurotrophic factors induced under cerebral ischemia are brain-derived neurotrophic factor (BDNF), basic fibroblast growth factor (bFGF), glial cell line-derived neurotrophic fader (GDNF), nerve growth factor (NGF), transfoming growth factor (TGF-β1), etc.

Although neurotrophic factors such as factors as mentioned above under cerebral ischemia are endogenously induced, in reality, the ischemic tissue of the brain is hardly rescued sufficiently, and the ability to synthesize protein is extremely reduced due to impaired energy metabolism. The effect of endogenous neurotrophic factors is insufficient because sufficient amount of neurotrophic factor is not synthesized from mRNA. Therefore, exogenous administration of a large amount of neurotrophic factors has been attempted to rescue brain ischemic tissue (Sato M, et al: Arzneimittel Forshung 35:790, 1985) (Skaper SD, et al: Methods Mol Biol 1727:1,2018). Experimentally, GNDF showed the strongest neuroprotective effect, followed by neurotrophin-3 (NT-3), vascular endothelial growth factor (VEGF), and insulin-like growth factor (IGF-1).

§20 Ischemic tolerance

Environmental stress are heat shock, active oxygen, hyperosmolarity, ultraviolet light, radiation, and viral infection. The brain can acquire resistance to ischemia by applying stress to the body for a very short time. The ischemic tolerance phenomenon caused by various preconditioning stresses can suppress ischemic neuronal cell death (Kitagawa T, et al : Brain Research: 528:21, 1990) (Kitagawa T, et al :Rinsho Shinkeigaku 39:1291,1999 in Japanese). However, it takes about 24 hours to acquire ischemic tolerance.

If the ischemic attack is not too strong, neurons show various protective responses triggered by intracellular Ca rise and free radical production. A typical example is the expression of stress proteins such as heat shock proteins (Hsp70, HsP72). It is expressed when exposed to various stresses such as heat, chemical substances, ischemia, hypoglycemia, hypoxia, chronic ischemia, and other oxidative stresses, binds to synthesized proteins, and regulates protein folding and unfolding. It repairs by functioning as a molecular chaperone to control folding and unfolding. A chaperone is a type of HSP that regulates protein folding. Oxygen Regulated Protein 150 (ORP150) is a substance similar to heat shock proteins, and is a general term for stress proteins that occur when the oxygen concentration in the surrounding environment of cells decreases. Stress proteins that occur in a hypoglycemic environment are called glucose regulated proteins (GRPs).

Proteins that cannot be repaired undergo ubiquitination and are transported to an enzyme complex called the proteasome where they are degraded. Consequently, damage is reduced to ischemic nerve tissue.

Folding disease is the accumulation of defective proteins in cells due to abnormalities in the folding process. This includes Alzheimer's disease and Parkinson's disease. In addition, manganese-SOD(Mn-SOD), which is an antioxidant enzyme, and Bcl-2, which is an apoptosis suppressor gene, are also involved in the ischemic tolerance phenomenon (Kirino T, et al: J Cereb Blood Flow Metab 22:1283, 2002).

Remote ischemic conditioning is a phenomenon in which, for example, complete ischemia of the lower extremities (manchette 200 mm HG, 4 times for 5 minutes) is performed during cerebral ischemia, the collateral circulation on the brain surface expands and the infarction shrinks. Akt-eNOS, one of signal transduction system, is involved in vascular endothelial cells. For remote ischemic conditioning, the same phenomenon occurs not only in cerebral infarction but also in myocardial infarction.

The above-mentioned chaperone is a general term for proteins that bind to unfolded (denatured) proteins and help them to be properly folded (native state). Folding is the process by which proteins acquire proper structure and normal function, and chaperones assist in this process. Chaperones are released from the substrate after folding is completed and do not become part of the substrate after folding. Moreover, the structure of the chaperone does not change before and after the reaction, and the structure after folding is not specified.

§21 Reperfusion injury

If 10-12 ml of CBF is maintained, reperfusion is imperfectly reversible. If it is below this level, it causes an increase in excitatory amino acids, membrane depolarization, lipid peroxidation, ROS generation, and an increase in intracellular Ca concentration. Pathologically, it can be rescued by reperfusion if it is at the stage of neuron microvacuolation.

When reperfusion occurs, the mechanism of brain cell injury associated with reperfusion is that activated neutrophils release various inflammatory factors, and cell adhesion factors are activated. Activation of various enzymatic systems and non-enzymatic cell damage progresses due to the increase in intracellular Ca concentration after ischemia. The ability to synthesize protein may already be damaged by ischemia, but the degree of damage depends on the ischemia resistance of the ischemic tissue. Spontaneous recanalization occurs in 20% of cases within 24 hours and 80% within 1 week of middle cerebral artery embolism (Fieschi C, et al : J Neurol Sci 91:311, 1989) (Wardlaw J, et al : Stroke 23:1826,1992) (Zanette E, et al : Stroke 26:430,1995). Hemorrhagic infarction occurs even with spontaneous recanalization, but there are few fatal major hemorrhages centered on the basal ganglia, and most of them are small hemorrhages in the cerebral cortex and white matter with few neurological deficits caused by recirculation. However, when thrombectomy or revascularization is actively performed, this phenomenon may often occur to a higher degree, and at least the outcome that surpasses this natural course must be brought about. Regardless of whether spontaneous recanalization or intentional recanalization is involved, treatment of cerebral ischemia cannot be considered if the recanalization phenomenon were ignored.

Ischemia cannot be considered ignoring reperfusion injury. The existence of reperfusion injury has come to be recognized in animal experiments, since the tissue injury in the reperfusion model is more severe than that in the permanent ischemia model. When the perfusion pressure during reperfusion is low, microcirculatory disturbance is caused, infarct expansion is promoted, and blood cell components accumulate in blood vessels, causing failure at the capillary level, which is called capillary plugging.

Summary of post-reperfusion course:

1. Due to the resumption of blood flow after cerebral ischemia, CBF transiently becomes excessive than normal (postischemic hyperperfusion), then gradually decreases, and coupling between metabolism and cerebral blood flow is established, resulting in a decrease below normal (postischemic hypoperfusion).
2. With the resumption of blood flow, oxygen flows into the ischemic lesion, and tissue damage progresses due to increased production of ROS at the site of ischemic injury.
3. Ca influx activates Ca-dependent enzymes such as calpain and proteolytic enzymes, resulting in tissue damage.
4. Vasogenic edema occurs due to the influx of Na, H_20 and macromolecular proteins such as albumin.
5. Glucose influx activates anaerobic glycolysis, and the lactic acid produced promotes acidosis.
6. Blood components such as platelets, leukocytes, and fibrinogen adhere and aggregate to various adhesion molecules that are upregulated under cerebral ischemia, resulting in production of thrombi and secondary microcirculatory disorders such as the no-reflow phenomenon.
7. Inflammatory cells such as leukocytes and macrophages infiltrate into tissues from blood vessels, and various cytokines, free radicals, proteolytic enzymes, etc. produced in inflammatory cells promote tissue damage. Along with those, up-regulation of various cell adhesion factors in vascular endothelial cells, tissue damage due to

tissue migration of macrophages, etc., exacerbation of inflammation promotes vasogenic edema.

§22 Expression of HMGB1 in ischemia

In the early stages of ischemia, nuclear histone-derived high mobility group box 1 (HMGB1) is released extracellularly from neurons in the cerebral cortex penumbra and ischemic center due to nuclear collapse, and induces inflammatory response and cell death. HMGB1 is released from the activated macrophage, monocyte and necrotic cell by stimuli such as TNF-α, IL-1β, and LPS (lipopolysaccharide; it is like endotoxin, and it activates macrophages), which are synthesized in the initial reaction of inflammation. As mentioned above, it is actively released by these stimuli from the activated macrophage and monocyte, or released from necrotic cells. In active release, HMGB1 is acetylated and phosphorylated to control its translocation into the nucleus, while it is secreted out of the cell by secretory lysosomes.

After translocating from the nucleus to the cytoplasm, HMGB1 is immediately released outside the cells, and HMGB1 acts as an upstream signal initiator not only in the brain but throughout the body in the early stages of inflammatory reactions. The proinflammatory action of HMGB1 alone is weak, and is significantly enhanced in the presence of other factors such as IL-1, IL-6, IL-17, IL-23, TNF-α and LPS. Although the administration of anti-HMGB1 antibody has been experimentally shown to reduce infarct size, it has not been applied clinically.

In 1999, the usefulness of HMGB1 as a lethal mediator of sepsis as a severity marker and therapeutic target substance was highlighted. HMGB1 released extracellularly activates NFκB through interactions with receptors for advanced glycation end products (RAGE) existing on various cell membranes, and induces inflammatory reactions and apoptosis. HMGB1 itself has inflammatory and cytotoxic effects, and extracellularly released HMGB1 directly affects sourrounding peripheral cells, resulting in ischemia/reperfusion, sepsis, acute lung injury, trauma, postoperative, and diffuse intravascular coagulation. It causes not only acute inflammation, but also pathological conditions such as chronic inflammation such as rheumatoid arthritis, arteriosclerosis, and so on.

Conversely, after interaction between HMGB1 and RAGE on the cell membrane, signal transduction into the cell has been reported to activate the NFκB signaling pathway in macrophages and neutrophils through phosphorylation of MAPKs.

§23 If a diabetes patient develops a cerebral infarction:

In diabetes, excess sugar in the blood binds to advanced glycation end product (AGE), and AGE binds to RAGE, causing damage to cells with the receptors (retina, nerve cells, vascular endothelial cells, etc.). HMGB1 is released from neurons in the early stages of ischemic brain injury. In addition to the action of various cytokines, an inflammatory reaction is induced, causing a vicious circle, and extracellular HMGB1 increases, becoming a factor exacerbating ischemic brain damage in diabetic conditions, and severe inflammatory reactions occur not only in the ischemic center but also in the penumbra. Finally they will cause cell death.

It is closely related to AGEs, which are non-enzymatic peroxidation products caused by oxidative stress on proteins, lipids, and nucleic acids by free radicals. NFκβ activates the AGE-responsive RAGE, and ROS induced by hyperglycemia increases the expression of HMGB1 and RAGE.

In addition, hyperglycemia activates lipoxygenase (LPX) and cyclooxygenase (COX) in the arachidonic acid cascade, leading to the production of various prostaglandins with platelet-aggregating action. In short, if a diabetic patient develops a cerebral infarction, it will be more severe than a normal cerebral infarction. In diabetic patients with hyperglycemia, the metabolic environment of the brain after reperfusion is worse than in ischemic stroke in normal blood sugar conditions. As a cause, in addition to oxidative stress accelerated by hyperglycemia, the NO-derived obstacle mechanism acts. One is the production of peroxynitrite anion, and the subsequent production of ROS such as hydroxyl radicals exacerbates the situation.

Oxidative stress is markedly elevated during diabetes. The following (1) to (6) are thought to be the mechanisms of oxidative stress production during diabetes.

(1) Reducing sugars such as glucose non-enzymatically form Schiff bases with amino groups of proteins, then

form stable Amadori compounds by Amadori rearrangement, and active oxygen is generated in the process of self-oxidation of these compounds.

(2) After that, irreversible dehydration and condensation are repeated to form AGEs. When AGEs bind to AGE receptors present on endothelial cells, they promote the production of ROS, activate NF-κβ as a transcription factor, promote the secretion of various cytokines and growth factors, and induce inflammatory reactions. In chronic hyperglycemic conditions such as diabetes, AGEs are progressively formed and accumulated in circulating blood and tissues, increasing oxidative stress.

(3) In hyperglycemia, the polyol metabolic pathway is activated and glucose is converted to fructose. Since fructose has a stronger action to saccharify proteins than glucose, the production of ROS is further enhanced, and coupled with the consumption of NADPH accompanying polyol metabolism and the resulting decrease in glutathione reductase. Consequently, intracellular oxidative stress is increased and disability of cell functions occurs.

(4) Activation of protein kinase C (PKC) enhances the NADPH oxidase activity of vascular cells and enhances the production of oxidative stress.

(5) AGEs reduce the activity of antioxidant enzymes such as SOD and GPx, as well as the content of low molecular weight antioxidant factors such as glutathione, vitamin C and vitamin E.

(6) The reaction between superoxide anion (O_2-) and NO produces peroxynitrite (ONOO-), which has a strong nitrating effect, and nitrates proteins.

§24 Nicotinamide adenine dinucleotide phosphate (NADPH)

It is a substance that appears in the glycolysis system of internal respiration. It is used for transfer of hydrogen and electrons (oxidation and reduction) and a coenzyme for dehydrogenase. A coenzyme is a non-protein low-molecular organic compound that expresses the activity of an enzyme. It is synthesized by pentose phosphate pathway (PPP) as described below, and it is a carrier of electrons and hydrogen. The electron transport chain is one of the three systems (glycolysis, citric acid cycle, electron transport chain) for making ATP, and most of ATP is made in the electron transport chain. NADPH is synthesized in the PPP. NADH is mainly used in the TCA cycle and mitochondrial electron transport system. NADH is generally used in catabolic reactions and NADPH in anabolic reactions.

Pentose phosphate pathway (PPP)

Glutathione and glutathione peroxidase play a central role in elimination of ROS in the brain, and reduced glutathione is essential for this reaction. Glutathione becomes oxidized upon removal of H_2O_2 and reduced in the presence of NADPH. Supplying NADPH is the main important action of PPP. That is, PPP, which is a glycolytic bypass of glucose metabolism, does not contribute to ATP production, but is important in reducing oxidative stress by producing NADPH, and is generated in the brain that continues to oxidatively metabolize large amounts of glucose. PPP is involved in elimination of ROS.

§25 Dynamics of Ca ions in reperfusion injury

Intraneuronal Ca influx through NMDA-type glutamate receptors causes neuronal injury. NMDA-type glutamate receptors have subtypes. NMDA receptors with the NR2A subunit act neuroprotectively, while NMDA receptors with the NR2B subunit act neuropathically. As for downstream signaling, elevated Ca concentration activates CaMK1/4 (Ca calmodulin kinase) and induces downstream neuroprotective factors by activating CREB (a factor that regulates gene expression).

Mitochondrial dysfunction and reperfusion

Mitochondria (Mt) contain many enzymes that produce ATP, but all of them are inactivated by ischemia. Inactivation of cytochrome oxidase and MnSOD, in particular, prevents effective utilization of oxygen during reperfusion and produces excessive amounts of ROS, resulting in progression of Mt membrane damage. As a result, the respiratory chain is damaged and unsaturated fatty acid peroxidation occurs, releasing Ca stored in the Mt into the cytoplasm.

Changes in the ischemic center are such that if the preceding focal cerebral ischemia lasts for about 2 hours, the Mt respiratory chain function is rapidly restored by reperfusion, but it is subsequently damaged secondary by ROS and free radicals.

Damage to the complex (described later) and increased intracellular Ca concentration after reperfusion are the causes of brain damage derived from Mt. Apoptosis is induced by activation of protease, nuclease and phospholipase caused by increase of intracellular Ca concentration.

A phenomenon called membrane permeability transition (MPT) is involved in Ca influx into Mt and may cause neuronal death (Hunter P, et al: Arch Biochem Biophys 195:468,1979). In other words, this is a mechanism called permeability transition pore (PTP) or Mt membrane permeabilization (MMP), which is a phenomenon in which the permeability of the Mt inner membrane increases in a Ca-dependent manner. MPT is regulated by cyclophilin D (Cyp-D). Excessive Ca concentration within Mt causes the production of ROS followed by neuronal death.

MPT is caused by disturbance of an ion channel from the outer membrane to the inner membrane of Mt. The complex (channel), which causes MPT, consists of adenine nucleotide transporter (ANT) on the inner membrane side, voltage-dependent anion channel (VDAC) on the outer membrane side, and Cyp-D in the matrix of Mt. Normally, VDAC and ANT come into contact and combine in the membrane lumen of Mt, forming a VDAC/ANT complex (intermembrane junctional coupling). Cyp-D in the matrix binds to ANT in a Ca-dependent manner, and further binds to the above complex to form a three-part Cyp-D/ANT/VDAC complex, which forms the center of the pore. It is thought that the opening of PTP is actually caused by the deformation of this complex (Crompton M, et al: J physiol 529:11, 2000). When oxidative stress occurs during reperfusion or when Ca concentration in Mt increases, PTP opening occurs and releases a large amount of apoptosis-inducing proteins such as cytochrome C, apoptosis-inducing factor, and caspase into the cytoplasm. Bcl-2 protein controls the acceleration of the opening of MPT. By the opening, cytochrome C, which was released into cytoplasm, activates caspase cascade. This opening is suppressed by cyclosporin A, etc.

An electron transport system exists in the Mt. This function is reduced by ischemia, but is completely restored by reperfusion if the degree and duration of ischemia is mild. However, when the degree and duration of ischemia become high, reperfusion instead destroys the electron transport function, and this phenomenon is the enlargement of the PTP. In this mechanism, the Mt Ca concentration, which was elevated during ischemia, returns to normal by reperfusion, but it soon rises and opens the PTP, interacting with the generation of pro-oxidants in the peroxidized state.

§26 Metabolism in mitochondria

Mt occupy 40% of the cell's volume and 90% of ROS occur in Mt. In organella, the largest amount of Ca is stored in the endoplasmic reticulum, followed by large amounts in Mt (Fig.3). The Mt membrane has an outer membrane and an inner membrane, and the membrane is made of "phospholipids." The area surrounded by the inner membrane is the matrix, the inner membrane of the outer membrane is the inner limiting membrane, and the part invaginated into the matrix is the cristae. Furthermore, aerobic respiration is carried out in a structure called the intermembrane space (the figure below), which is surrounded by the outer membrane and the inner limiting membrane. The "citric acid cycle" takes place in the Mt "matrix," but the place where the "electron transport system" reactions take place is the Mt "inner membrane."

In Mt, there are the following three systems in the reaction for producing adenosine phosphate (ATP): 1. glycolysis, 2. citric acid cycle, 3. electron transport chain. Among them, the electron transport chain produces the

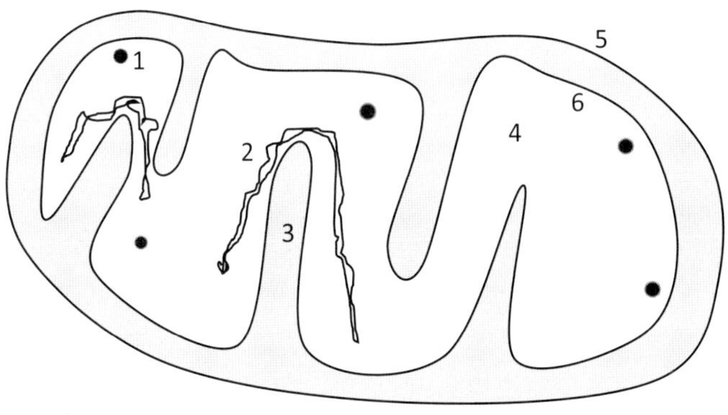

Fig.3. Schematic drawing of cross section of a mitochondrion: (1) ribosome, (2) mitochondrial DNA, (3) cristae, (4) matrix, (5) outer membrane, (6) inner membrane.

largest amount of ATP. A large amount of 36 ATP is produced (the amount of ATP produced differs depending on the organ), and most of the ATP is produced by the electron transport system. In other words, the electron transport system is a system for efficiently producing ATP from "NADH+H+ and FADH2" produced in the glycolysis and citric acid cycle.

First, in glycolysis, NADH is finally utilized for ATP synthesis through oxidative phosphorylation by glycolysis of glucose by glycolysis. This reaction takes place in the cytoplasm rather than in Mt. 1 mol of glucose produces 2 mol of pyruvate or lactate, in the process consuming 2 mol of ATP and producing 4 mol of ATP. This results in 2 moles of ATP.

Next, in the citric acid cycle (progressing within the mitochondrial matrix) pyruvate is then metabolized via acetyl-CoA, allowing pyruvate to cross the outer and inner Mt membranes without difficulty. Incidentally, NADH+H+ is also created in the process of converting pyruvate to acetyl-CoA.

Next, in the electron transport chain (progressing in the inner membrane of Mt), a large amount of ATP is synthesized here by consuming NADH and $FADH_2$ obtained in the glycolysis and citric acid cycle. In this electron transport system, electrons are transported along the order of the complex (it is called a "complex" because it has a complicated structure. "Respiratory chain complex," "Enzyme complex," "Protein complex" are also the same). Complexes are numbered I, II, III, IV, and V, shown below.

Complex I: NADH: ubiquinone oxidoreductase complex, Complex II: succinate dehydrogenase complex, Complex III: ubiquinol: cytochrome c reductase complex, Complex IV: cytochrome c oxidase complex, Complex V: ATP synthase.

Hydrogen's "electrons (e-)" move through this "complex" of I to IV, and the "electrons" are relayed (transmitted) to complexes I to IV embedded in the membrane, and finally becomes water. Then, ATP is synthesized with the energy when "protons (H^+)" in the intermembrane space move to the matrix through "complex V." In other words, the electron transport system forms a proton gradient (H^+ concentration gradient) across the Mt inner membrane in the process in which electrons emitted from NADH and FADH2 are transferred in the Mt inner membrane, and by the proton driving force system it produces ATP from ATP synthase. In other words, ATP production begins when NADH+H+ and FADH2 produced in the glycolytic system and the citric acid cycle are transported to the inner membrane of Mt.

What is mitochondrial stress?

When exposed to excessive stress, the Mt of cells suffer from various disorders such as overproduction of ROS, damage to Mt DNA, and accumulation of defective proteins in the matrix. This can lead to apoptosis and necrosis (Mt unfolded protein response).

PLA2 and free radicals impair the functions of receptor ion channel constituent proteins and phospholipids due to ischemia-induced Ca elevation in neurons, resulting in a sustained increase in Ca, and Mt dysfunction due to Ca uptake into Mt leading to apoptosis and necrosis. Mt dysfunction occurs when the acidity of ROS and Ca uptake in Mt exceeds thresholds and MPT pore opening is induced.

The Mt outer membrane has a high chemotaxis permeability, and cytoplasmic Ca easily enters the intermembrane space. Ca in this intermembrane space is transported to the matrix by Ca uniporters in the inner membrane utilizing the H+ electrochemical concentration gradient. Ca transport to the matrix is activated when the cytosolic Ca concentration exceeds a certain set point. The endoplasmic reticulum has similar functions, but to a lesser extent than Mt. Since the rate (velocity) of releasing Ca out of the cell is slow, the Ca concentration in the matrix continues to rise, and when it exceeds a certain level, Mt dysfunction begins. Pore formation, ROS production, etc. occur, inner membrane cytochrome C is released from the PTP into the cytoplasm, and the apoptotic cascade (caspase cascade) is activated. The absolute amount of Ca in Mt is related to cell death. Mt PTP opening increases not only ROS but also RNS. Bcl-2 protein regulates the promotion of PTP opening. Cytochrome C, released into the cytoplasm by this opening, activates the caspase cascade.

Concerning Mt electron transport system and NADPH/$NADP^+$ ratio and redox, "oxidation occurs when oxygen is received, and reduction occurs when hydrogen or electrons are received." NADPH is the reduced form and

NADP+ is the oxidized form. Therefore, when the ratio of NADPH/NADP$^+$ is large, it means that the ratio of the reduced form is large. That is, reduction is dominant (oxidative stress is low). Conversely, when this value is low, it is under oxidative stress. The same is true for glutathione, which is used to reduce NADPH. Since the reduced form is GSH and the oxidized form is GSSG, the larger the GSH/GSSG ratio, the lower the oxidative stress in the cell. Concerning antioxidants combating oxidative stress, redox means reduction-oxidation, or oxidoreduction.

§27 Changes in protein synthesis ability and intracellular signaling system caused by reperfusion

Recovery of protein metabolism after resumption of blood flow takes about twice as long as the time until recovery of blood flow. Even in cells that recover blood flow early and escape cell death, their ability to synthesize proteins is markedly reduced.

In the normal condition, eukaryotic initiation factor (eIF) 2 is activated by another eIF (eIF2B) followed by the translation initiation. Both eIF2 and eIF2B are main translation initiation factors. Ribosomes start to initiate synthesizing proteins. When they initiate synthesizing, translation initiation factors such as eIF2B act in a coordinated manner.

However, endoplasmic reticulum stress is a rather complex story that begins with various stresses that occur in living organisms, such as viral infection, hypoglycemia, hypoxia, amino acid starvation, cerebral ischemia, heat shock, oxidative stress, and protein misfolding. The resulting abnormal proteins within the cell accumulate in the endoplasmic reticulum, and this series of mechanisms by which the endoplasmic reticulum tries to cope with the problem to prevent the cell from suffering major damage is called endoplasmic reticulum stress.

There are three response mechanisms for the unfolded protein response (UPR), which suppresses defective proteins caused by stress: 1. A pathway that suppresses mRNA translation and reduces the load by preventing new proteins from being delivered to the endoplasmic reticulum (for example, PERK). 2. Methods that increase folding capacity in the endoplasmic reticulum by inducing endoplasmic reticulum molecular chaperones such as glucose regulated protein 78 (GRP78) (e.g., IREI). 3. A pathway (such as ERAD) that enhance the ability of protein degradation mechanisms.

When eIF2α kinase (the following four types are molecules (enzymes) that catalyze eIF2α phosphorylation) detects stress, it is one of the mRNA translation initiation factors (protein synthesis initiation factors). It is eIF2α and phosphorylation occurs regardless of the type of stress. Under normal conditions, eIF2 is activated by another translation initiation factor, eIF2B, and has the effect of promoting translation initiation. Once protein synthesis begins, transcription initiation factors (e.g. eIF2B) work together. By the way, the four types of kinases mentioned above are PKR (double-stranded RNA dependent protein kinase), HRI (heme-regulated inhibitor), GCN2 (general control non-derepressible 2), and PERK (PKR-like endoplasmic reticulum kinase).

The above PERKs are activated by endoplasmic reticulum stress. That is, eIF2α is phosphorylated by the PERK cycle via PERK molecules, and inhibits the formation of protein synthesis complexes. It responds to various stress stimuli by suppressing or stopping protein synthesis.

First, the mechanism of translation termination is PERK. That is, BiP bound to PERK dissociates (see §5), forms a polymer of PERK, and is activated by phosphorylation. However, due to phosphorylation of eIF2α by PERK, the translation initiation complex cannot be formed, and intracellular mRNA translation is suppressed. If the UPR, which is the first step in endoplasmic reticulum stress, does not function properly, cells will die due to apoptosis.

More specifically, eIF2 is phosphorylated, and phosphorylated eIF2 binds to eIF2B in an unusual orientation, thereby inhibiting eIF2B activation, and phosphorylated eIF2 comes to act as an inhibitory factor for eIF2B (Kashiwagi K, et al: Science 10:1126,2010).

In areas of cerebral circulation disorders, when cells feel the stress of cerebral infarction or reperfusion, eIF2 is phosphorylated by eIF2B. EIF2 becomes a molecule that impairs the function of eIF2B. As a result, the activation of eIF2 is further attenuated by reperfusion, and transcription is suppressed.

Inositol requiring 1 (IRE1) dissociates from Bip and

becomes abundant, inducing chaperones, ERAD (described below), and factors that promote apoptosis.

Activating transcription factor 6 (ATF6) belongs to the CREB family of transcription factors involved in the induction of chaperone molecules.

If defective proteins cannot undergo UPR, they are folded by the calnexin cycle, but if that fails, they are transported back from the endoplasmic reticulum to the cytoplasm, ubiquitinated, and degraded by the proteasome. This phenomenon is called endoplasmic reticulum associated degradation (ERAD). PKR is a factor that detects viral RNA that has entered cells and exerts an antiviral effect, and phosphorylates eIF2α. HRI detects heme concentration and is activated by heme deficiency conditions and phosphorylates eIF2α. In addition to this, it is also activated by oxidative stress and heat shock. GCN2 phosphorylates eIF-2α in response to nutritional stress such as amino acid starvation.

Cell death induction pathway includes 1. A pathway mediated by the transcription factor c/EBP homologous protein (CHOP)/GADD153. 2. A pathway mediated by c-jun N-terminal kinase (JNK) through activation of TNF receptor-associated factor 2 (TRAF2). 3. If defective proteins are not reduced even after UPR, ERAD, and calnexin cycle, cells undergo apoptosis by caspases. There are three pathways mentioned above, and cell death is induced through one of them. Note that endoplasmic reticulum stress occurs not only in nerve cells but also in astrocytes. Activation of calpain by reperfusion causes protein synthesis disorder.

ROS are deeply involved in reaction pathways leading to apoptosis and necrosis in various cells. Signal transduction systems involving various PKs are involved in post-reperfusion neuronal injury, but these PKs are further regulated by ROS.

Cadherins, named after "calcium" and "adhere", are a group of glycoproteins that exist on the cell surface and are molecules that control cell adhesion. Ca are necessary for functional expression. It is protected from decomposition by protease under the presence of Ca.

Reperfusion activates NFκβ in the vascular endothelium and enhances neutrophil adhesion. In particular, ICAM-1 is expressed by the generated ROS. However, ICAM-1 is inactivated by endothelium-derived NO.

§28 ROS, NO, cytokines and in vivo antioxidant after reperfusion

IL-1β has a damaging effect, TNFα has a bilateral effect, and IL-6 has a protective effect on the early pathology after cerebral ischemia. Their origins are microglia for IL-1β, neurons and microglia for TNFα, and neurons for IL-6. The timing of onset is 12-24 hours after ischemia, which is prominent in the peri-ischemic area and may be associated with increased infarct size.

As to why ROS are the basis of the brain injury mechanism after reperfusion, firstly, oxygen radicals generated in the X/XO (xanthine/xanthine oxidase) pathway are the origin of the radical production system, and various ROS, NO, and ONOO- are formed. It is understood that these react with various signal transduction factors to cause peroxidation of membrane phospholipids, peroxidation of DNA, and inactivation of various enzymes.

NO generated from neurons is highly toxic, and excessive NO after reperfusion is closely related to the expansion of infarct lesions. The target of the disorder is the Mt. NO reacts with ROS to form N_2O_2, which produces various radicals, destroys the Mt electron transport system, and destroys proteins and lipids in the Mt themselves. It eventually leads to failure of PTP.

Brain tissue has traditionally been equipped with its own antioxidant functions. For example, they are GTX, glutathione reductase, catalase, and SOD. Ischemia impairs their function and leads to production of ROS in Mt following reperfusion.

Energy failure after ischemia and increased intracellular Ca concentration promote membrane phospholipid damage, and this situation is further aggravated after reperfusion by increasing ROS due to oxygenation followed by enhancing lipid peroxidation.

An important source of ROS production in reperfusion is:

1. Xanthine oxidase: ROS is produced from O_2 when hypoxanthine produced by catabolism of ATP during ischemia is converted to xanthine by xanthine oxygenase.
2. NADH oxygenase
3. Mt: Electrons leak when the electron transport system restarts due to reperfusion, and ROS is generated from O_2.
4. Endothelial NOs: Normally, eNOs binds to tetrahydro-

biopterin to produce NO. During reperfusion, tetrahydrobiopterin binds to NO synthase (which causes vasoconstriction) to produce ROS from O_2. Mt PTPs are normally closed, but are opened by excessive ROS or low ATP; then allows movement of large molecules between matrix and cytoplasm → Mt swelling, intracellular Ca increase → further opening of PTPs → followed by cell death.

Chapter 2 Dementia

Dementia

§1 What is dementia?

There are various types of dementia, but the most common is Alzheimer's disease (abbreviated as AD), which is the basis of dementia. Dementia is often discussed on the basis of symptoms of AD. It consists of core symptoms and peripheral symptoms. The symptoms are very diverse, complex, and difficult to understand.

Core symptoms (cognitive symptoms) are common symptoms that occur in any dementia when cognitive function declines: memory disorders, disorientation, executive dysfunction, complex attention disorders, language disorders, spatial cognitive disorders, etc. More specifically, they become forgetful (especially in recent memory), they make more mistakes in their efforts to maintain their attention and are slow to respond, they are unable to organize things well, and they are unable to perform movements smoothly. They become impossible to put the car in the garage with the back of the car, show decrease in vocabulary causing short sentences, need nursing care as it progresses, get lost their way when going out and become a problem for the police, get unable to remember the faces of family members who do not live together.

Peripheral symptoms, generally said behavioral and psychological symptoms (BPSD) of dementia, are symptoms that appear accompanying core symptoms (detailed in §5).

In Chapter 2, I will discuss the main causes of dementia (underlying diseases).

§2 Dementia and cognitive function

At first, I vaguely described the symptoms of dementia, but I am not diagnosing dementia only from these confused symptoms. There are various diagnostic criteria for diagnosing dementia, and representative ones are the International Classification of Diseases 10th edition (ICD-10) and the American Psychiatric Association DSM-5 (American psychiatric association. DSM-5, 2013).

To summarize the items common to each of these diagnostic criteria for dementia:

1. Learning and memory impairment (mainly recent episodic memory impairment, followed by time, place, and person in order).
2. Impaired executive function (planning, decision-making, etc.).
3. Linguistic disorders (names, words, fluency, grammar, syntax, etc.).
4. Complex attention disturbance (persistence, distribution, selectivity, processing speed).
5. Visuospatial cognitive impairment.
6. Social cognition (roughening of social behavior).

If we agree with two of these items, it is said to be dementia. In my ward, about 70% have dementia, and the average of Mini Mental State Examination (MMSE) of my patients is 17.4 (23 or less is dementia). People who meet one of these criteria are many among ordinary people.

In the first place, there may be an opinion that each of these criteria may be a cognitive dysfunction. It's very difficult to tell the difference, but are they really the same? In reality, the way of medical stuff's diagnosing (judgment) and understanding the pathophysiology changes depending on their background of the staff involved in the patient, that is:

a. Cognitive dysfunction specialists are not necessarily dementia specialists. Dementia experts are not experts in cognitive dysfunction.
b. Professionals working in disability support facilities do not know about dementia and see everything as an extension of developmental disorders.
c. Professionals working in nursing homes make anything dementia and cognitive dysfunction in the elderly associated with dementia.
d. Psychiatry ward makes the patient a mental illness.

This is something that is often said, and we should treat it with care. Also, even in my hospital, the barrier between experts in each field are high, and even if we hold a conference, it can be sometimes difficult to reach a compromise. However, in the case of dementia, it is salvation that a definitive diagnosis can be obtained by performing various tests such as imaging, cerebrospinal fluid, gene and blood tests.

So the question everyone has is what the difference between dementia and cognitive dysfunction is. Cognitive dysfunction is usually caused by the organic etiology of the cerebrum and includes cerebral focal symptoms such as aphasia, agnosia, and apraxia, attention disorders, memory disorders, judgment and problem-solving disorders, emotional disorders, executive dysfunction, and social behavioral abnormalities. Cognitive dysfunction is an administrative definition that does not include progressive diseases (although some may include progressive diseases such as malignant tumors) (Ministry of Health, Labor and Welfare, 2001).

Dementia is the persistent deterioration of cognitive functions (memory, language, recognition, executive function, etc.) across multiple areas due to acquired brain disorders (such as Alzheimer's disease) in people who have developed normally once. Patients with cognitive dysfunction (a broader concept than dementia) meet at least one of the diagnostic criteria for dementia. Anyway, difference includes confusing problems.

§3 General knowledge of dementia

Now for general knowledge about dementia:

In Japan, the number is 5 million and is on the rise: Increasing trend in Asia, decreasing trend in Europe.

Dementia is progressive. AD has a life expectancy of 12 years, and Lewy body dementia has a poor prognosis of 8 years. It is an organic rather than a functional disease (unlike schizophrenia). There is also early-onset dementia (under age 65), which is often hereditary. There are few genetic diseases in late onset dementia in general. Symptoms consist of core symptoms and peripheral symptoms called BPSD. Psychotherapy such as humanitude cannot improve the pathological changes in the brain, and the speed of progress does not change while transient amelioration of symptom can expected.

There is a FAST classification as a stage classification that expresses the severity of dementia (for example, as a notation of the III-3-9 degree system for consciousness disturbance), and it is easy to use. It is considered common sense that has gained general consensus. I would like you to know such things and proceed with the discussion. The table 1 shows the stages of progression in terms of symptoms in AD; it can be used as an evaluation criterion of another dementia and is simple. The table is revised from the original text, adding the MMSE for a reference (Table 1).

All dementias, with exceptions, are progressive, and exacerbation is seen during hospitalization (especially if hospitalized for a long period of time) or when a heavy burden is incurred. Except for special cases such as relocation damage, the overall flow shows gradual aggravation.

§4 Clinical course of dementia in the convalescent stage

I propose a figure of clinical course of dementia showing the fluctuation of FAST depending on the time, as shown in Fig.4. It is very easy to understand the fluctuation of FAST, but the dementia gradually progresses in spite of the recovery period.

The ordinate is severity, and the abscissa is time course. Since FAST (or FIM) for dementia patients has been on a downward slope since before the present illness, this line becomes further downward due to an present illness such as cerebral infarction. Complication such as systemic inflammatory response syndrome (SIRS) is added there, it will be considerably depressed. If the patient somewhat improves with treatment, as long-term hospitalization at an acute care hospital is rarely permitted, early discharge is encouraged and the patient is transferred to our hospital. In acute-stage, High-mobility group box-1 (HMGB-1) is released from necrotic tissue of cerebral infarction, or advanced glycation end product (AGE) caused by hyperglycemia binds to neuronal receptor for AGE in the presence of DM. Dementia is exacerbated by damaging nerve cells and impairing microglia, impairing the phagocytosis of amyloid β. Other than that, aspiration pneumonia, bacterial translocation, etc. occur. However, when he gets somewhat better, he is transferred to another hospital. What awaits after the transfer is relocation damage that occurs just after the transfer, which may include delirium followed by positive symptoms such as a desire to go home, falls from the bed, and falls in the hospital room. Attempts are made to improve the nutritional status, but the internal energy from the acute stage is large and a large amount of nutrition cannot be given, or tube feeding results in

Table1. Functional assessment staging (FAST)
(Sclan SG: Int Psychogeriatr: Functional assessment staging (FAST) in Alzheimer's disease: reliability, validity, and ordinality 4 Suppl 1:55,1992)

Stage	Stage Name	Characteristic	MMSE
1	Normal Aging	No deficit whatever	29-30
2	Possible Mild Cognitive Impairment	Subjective functional deficit	28-29
3	Mild Cognitive Impairment	Objective functional deficit interferes with a person's most complex tasks	24-28
4	Mild Dementia	IADLs become affected, such as bill paying, cooking, cleaning, travelling	19-20
5	Moderate Dementia	Needs help selecting proper attire	15
6a	Moderately Severe Dementia	Needs help putting on clothes	9
6b	Moderately Severe Dementia	Needs help bathing	8
6c	Moderately Severe Dementia	Needs help toileting	5
6d	Moderately Severe Dementia	Urinary incontinence	3
6e	Moderately Severe Dementia	Fecal incontinence	1
7a	Severe Dementia	Speaks 5-6 words during day	0
7b	Severe Dementia	Speaks only 1 word clearly	0
7c	Severe Dementia	Can no longer walk	0
7d	Severe Dementia	Can no longer sit up	0
7e	Severe Dementia	Can no longer smile	0
7f	Severe Dementia	Can no longer hold up head	0

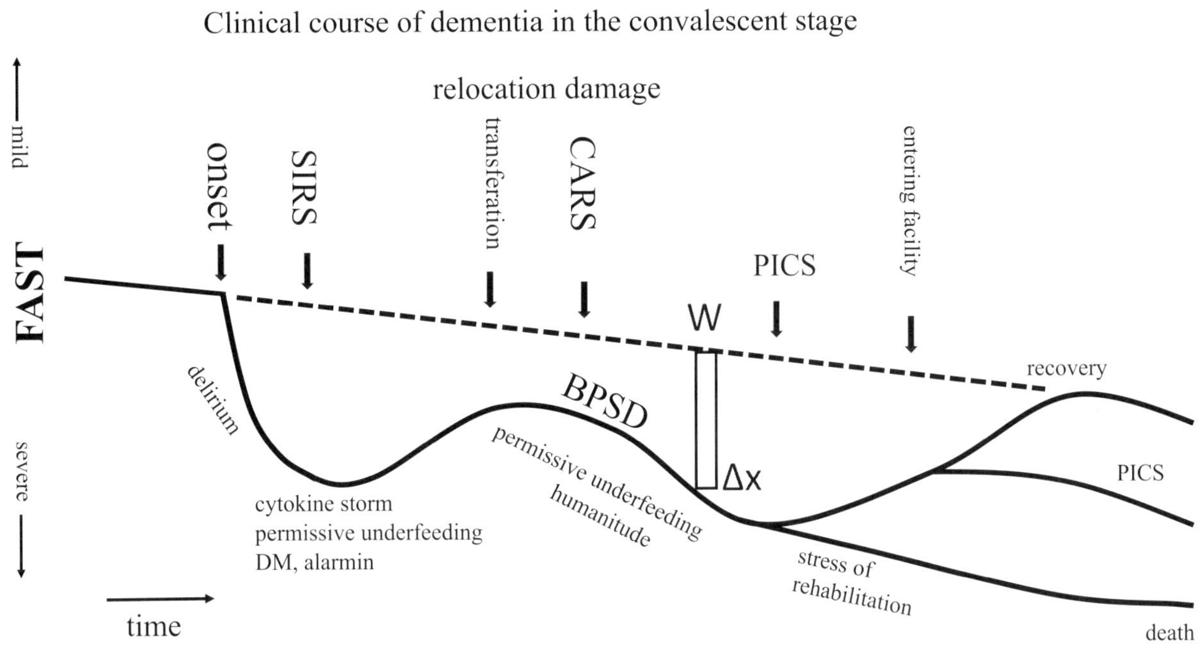

Fig.4. Clinical course of dementia in the convalescent stage, showing the fluctuation of FAST depending on the time. Ordinate shows FAST (severity of ADL caused by dementia), and abscissa is time course. Severity of dementia gradually progresses in spite of the recovery period through the fluctuation of FAST. The territory between the dotted line and real curve shows amount of rehabilitation exercise that the patient had to do for his original disease such as AD. The vertical bar in the figure is the work (joules) done in one day to improve the present state to the original better state.

excessive nutrition administration, which inevitably leads to permissive underfeeding.

I have no choice but to do humanitude in combination with rehabilitation for the descent of FAST. During this period, the patients may present with compensatory anti-inflammatory response syndrome (CARS), and we must be careful about infection and fever. In addition, post intensive care syndrome (PICS) also merged and the course became chaotic, and it was time to make decisions such as transferation to a facility, or a long-term care bed, and discharge at home. Family members are forced to make decisions about transferring critically ill patients, but I believe that the family is in PICS-F (detailed in §37) and cannot necessarily make the right decision, which is a terrible burden on the family. Curves representing these progressions are shown in Fig.4, which is a transition curve that I thought about based on our case. In the rounds of inpatients, it is always necessary to think about treatment while considering where the patient is on this curve.

Dementia is exacerbated by various diseases such as trauma, diabetes, and cerebral stroke if they are highly invasive. We investigated how much dementia (especially AD) was affected by femoral fracture in our convalescent ward. I investigated the functional outcome of 178 patients with femoral fractures, including 29 with co-existing AD in my ward. Of these, 12 patients (41%) had aggravated FAST even after rehabilitation and had difficulty in improving their function (become wheelchair users). The reason for this is thought to be that HMGB-1 released by tissue damage binds to receptor for AGE (RAGE) and damages to nerve cells, and damages to microglia which has phagocytosis of amyloid. Dementia is aggravated by increasing accumulation of amyloid β, which is the cause of AD, followed by formation of nucleotide binding-oligomerization domain-like receptor P3 (NLRP3) inflammasome (Sato M, et al : J Hyogo Medical Association 63: 44, 2020) .

The dotted line in the figure indicates that if the patient had not suffered a stroke, he would have been able to lead a peaceful daily life but he had to do rehabilitation. The vertical bar in the Fig.4 shows the work (joules) done in one day to improve (return) to his original FAST status.

§5 Peripheral symptoms of dementia

So what are peripheral symptoms (behavioral and psychological symptoms of dementia, 'BPSD')? As mentioned above, BPSD appear in association with core symptoms. These symptoms are influenced by genetic background, neuropathological findings in the brain, biochemical changes, psychological factors, social factors, environmental factors, etc. Individual differences are large due to these impacts. To put it simply, BPSDs show various variations depending on the person's personality, the environment in which they were born and raised, and the underlying disease of dementia. The concept of BPSD was proposed at the 7th International Geriatric Psychiatry Conference in 1995.

What kind of BPSD do you know? BPSD is classified into two: positive symptoms and negative symptoms. Positive symptoms are a general term for symptoms that make you feel that something is not there. It is a highly visible or audible symptom and accounts for 52% of BPSD. Specifically, in addition to the above auditory hallucinations and delusions, irritability, we usually include restlessness, abusive language, aggressive behavior such as resistance to nursing care, day-night reversal (sleep disorder, delirium), wandering, leaving the hospital, desire to return home, things taken delusions and groping. Negative symptoms are a general term that means that what is originally there is lost, and the basic symptoms are autism and emotional dullness. Negative symptoms include lack of emotion, low motivation, anxiety, depression, apathy, impatience, not pressing the nurse call (no matter how many times I explain it, the patient can't understand the meaning or importance), urinary and fecal incontinence, refusal of rehabilitation, irritability, loss of dentures (throwing them away by themselves), etc. They are serious for the person himself and are well expressed in Sawako Ariyoshi's novel in 1972 "The twilight years (ecstatic person)."

Other than those, there are neither negative nor positive symptoms. There are peculiar symptoms depending on the causative disease of dementia. Examples include eating behavior disorders (overeating, pica behavior, sweet food preference), stereotyped behavior, shoplifting, socially inappropriate behavior, and leaving behavior, delusions of being stolen, coprophilia, sexual harassment, wandering, REM sleep behavior disorder, twilight syndrome (ward stuffs have often experienced that they are busy from evening to midnight in the ward because of this), hallucinations (for example, insects are crawling, children are visible, strangers live in their own house, the wife is fake), and so on. Staffs are battling these BPSDs every day.

Mechanism of psychiatric symptoms

In some occasions such as antipsychotic drugs have to be administered we must be aware of the effects and adverse events. In general, the mechanisms of the appearance of psychotic symptoms, which may be associated with psychosis, effects or adverse events induced by antipsychotic drugs, the following circuits are emphasized, although not all BPSDs are easily associated with some pathways (Fig.5).

1. Positive symptoms such as hallucinations and delusions appear due to hyperactivity of dopamine D2 receptors in the midbrain-limbic pathway.
2. Negative symptoms appear due to decreased dopamine levels in the midbrain cortical system. It is related to depression.
3. Extrapyramidal symptom (EPS) appears due to dopamine D2 receptor blockade in the nigrostriatal pathway.
4. Hypothalamic D2 receptor blockade causes prolactin (PRL) elevation (infertility in women).

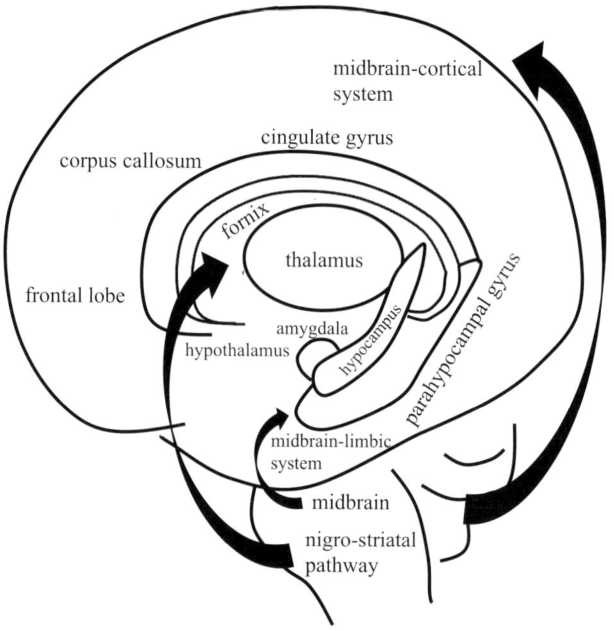

Fig.5. Simple schema of several pathways showing mechanism of action of antipsychotics.

5. Disturbances in the dorsolateral prefrontal cortex of the frontal lobe (executive function), lateral orbital cortex (personality change, disinhibition), and anterior cingulate cortex (apathy).

Schneider's first-class symptoms

Although slightly different from the symptoms described above, symptoms somewhat related to BPSD include Schneider's first-class symptoms. These are symptoms that form the basis of the diagnosis of schizophrenia, especially the positive symptoms, but they are partly similar to BPSD of dementia. That is;

Thought echoing: The patients can hear what he is thinking as an auditory hallucination or other person can get to know what he is thinking.

Auditory hallucinations of multiple people in conversational form: The patients can hear multiple people are gossiping about him in conversational form. He can hear the conversation as auditory hallucination.

Auditory hallucinations in the form of criticism of one's own actions: The patient can hear voices condemning his own actions or words.

Malicious acts on the body: The patient is convinced that someone is watching him 24 hours a day, or that someone is trying to kill him.

Thought stealing: The patient feels that someone else is stealing his thoughts.

Interference with thoughts: The patient feels that his thoughts are being interfered with by others.

Thought propagation: The patient feels that his thoughts are leaked to those around him.

Delusional perception: The patient thinks forcibly linking unrelated things.

Manipulative experience: The patient feels that someone else is manipulating his thoughts, intentions, and actions.

§6 Diseases that are difficult to differentiate from dementia

1. Age-related cognitive decline (ARCD): a decline in cognitive performance due to age.
2. Mild cognitive impairment (MCI): It meets only one definition of dementia and includes a decline in cognitive performance rather than a decline due to age.
3. Mental ageing (mentioned below).
4. Geriatric depression: Self-awareness of memory disturbance (but exaggerated) and seriousness, hypochondrial delusions (convincing him that he has a serious illness though he is not sick), delusions of poverty, and depressed mood. Antidepressants are effective.
5. Delirium: Sudden onset with disturbance of consciousness, but transiently followed by recovery. Note that the presence of delirium does not imply dementia, but it is often the beginning of dementia.
6. Late-onset paraphrenia (described later).
7. Schizophrenia: It may be due to high levels of dopamine D2 in the mesolimbic system. Pathophysiological state is often similar to dementia. Medical treatment is similar.

The above pathologies should be precisely distinguished from dementia. In my ward, other than dementia, there are many 1~5 of the above.

Mental ageing

Mental ageing is not dementia but much like dementia. It has following characteristics.

1. Age-related changes (older), not dementia (albeit difficult to distinguish).
2. Memory decline (word recall disorder, forgetfulness). Benign forgetfulness (dementia is malignant forgetfulness).
3. Emotional changes → Flattening of emotion, less emotional, weakening of will and desire.
4. Personality change → Conservative, self-centered, irritable, short-tempered, loyal, roundabout, sharpened or maturing.

Though it is not a psychiatric disorder, the mental state and behavior of elderly people may differ slightly from that of young people. He is vigorous and has a bright side that young people cannot match regardless of age, but it is likely to be in the manner of an old person. These are called mental ageing.

Late paraphrenia

This concept was first described by Roth of England in 1955 (Roth M, et al: J Mental Science 101: 281, 1955), and is one of the diseases that are difficult to distinguish from dementia. For example; Single middle-aged and elderly women with deafness and social isolation present "Mr. A in the neighborhood is talking bad about me" "The upper floor is noisy" with symptoms such as sudden-onset delusions of persecution, delusions of grandeur, and auditory hallucinations.

The concept of late onset schizophrenia-like psychosis (LOSLP) had been proposed for late paraphrenia and included in schizophrenia (Howard R, et al: Am J Psychiatry 152:172,2000). In other words, this type of disease, which develops after the age of 40, has come to be considered a type of schizophrenia. Its symptoms are single middle-aged and elderly women, deafness, social isolation, immigration and other risk factors, low genetic component, lack of disease awareness, general elderly with preserved cognitive function and ADLs. The incidence of dementia is higher than that of the elderly. Troubles with neighbors, refusal to receive treatment, exclusion from the community, living in a poor environment in a garbage house, intense delusions about specific neighbors, and sometimes visual and auditory hallucinations (infrequently).

Should we consider these as prodromal symptoms of dementia, or schizophrenia of late onset? There are many cases of refusal to go to the hospital, and the progress is difficult to understand.

§7 Current concept (classification) of schizophrenia

Currently, the concept of schizophrenia is classified into the following three categories, but there may be a little controversial (Howard R,et al: Am J Psychiatry 152:172,2000).

1. Early-onset schizophrenia (EOS): Onset in young adulthood. Same as schizophrenia so far. Etiology is abnormal dopamine D2 in the mesolimbic system, chromosome 5 abnormality, synaptic abnormality, etc.
2. Late-onset schizophrenia (LOS): Late-onset schizophrenia with onset at age 40 or older.
3. Very-late-onset schizophrenia-like psychosis (VLOSLP): a new category which was separated from late paraphrenia.

VLOSLP occurs after age 60. It is the third most common mental illness among the elderly, after dementia and depression. There is little inheritance, there are quite a few patients who transition to dementia (easy to transition), and EOS sometimes transitions to dementia, but less frequently than VLOSLP. It is characterized by a delusion called "partition delusion" (someone comes in through the wall). Pathologically, argyrophilic grain dementia often presents with VLOSLP. Treatment is started with aripiprazole and effective in a third of patients (i.e. slightly less effective). It is common in women. Hypersensitivity to antipsychotics is sometimes observed. Families are often exhausted by the patient's symptom.

Symptoms of LOS and VLOSLP are sometimes similar to those of dementia. For example, when elderly patients with femoral fractures, lumbar fractures, or strokes are hospitalized, they often develop mental symptoms such as delirium and hallucinations, and we become unable to know the difference between schizophrenia and dementia. It is difficult to see the relationship between schizophrenia and dementia, but dementia may have characteristic radiological findings of each causative disease, and schizophrenia does not have them in principle.

Over time, LOS and VLOSLP may come to belong to one of the dementia diseases, and even if they are initially thought to be just early stages of dementia, they may come to belong to the diagnosis of schizophrenia over time.

Pathogenesis of schizophrenia

As a cause of schizophrenia (there are various hypotheses, but the following is one of them as an interesting mechanism), "the scrap & build hypothesis." The number of synapses is the highest in the first year after birth, and then decreases to about half of the peak at the age of 10. In other words, during the developmental stage of the brain, excessive circuits are created, from which necessary circuits are selected and strengthened, and unnecessary circuits are eliminated. This period is called the critical period, when the neural circuits are highly sensitive to the environment. Hypothesis that autism, schizophrenia, and dementia are scrap-and-build imbalances, or namely scrap-and-build diseases.

By the way, the onset of schizophrenia is 16-25 years old (25 people/100,000 people), followed by 46-55 years old (10 people/100,000 people). It increases at older than 65 years old (15 people/100,000 people). There are more females than males. Patients aged older than 40 years are characterized by a low frequency of family history, high educational attainment, and female gender. In LOS and VLOSLP, frontotemporal atrophy is very pronounced.

Relationship between schizophrenia and dementia

So how do we see the relationship between schizophrenia and dementia? Psychiatry has developed by classifying functional aspects (symptoms) for convenience, but with the recent development of medicine it is possible to explain (theoretically) materially (through examinations) well (recently, not only organic diseases but also functional diseases such as psychosis, investigations of functional imaging are being developed).

Schizophrenia, which has been thought of as a functional disease, and dementia, which assumes an organic disorder, sometimes show similar phenotypes, with similar symptoms and some overlapping pathologies. This is somehow an unsolved problem in neurological diseases.

The relationship between Alzheimer's disease and amyloid, schizophrenia and the dopamine hypothesis (relationship between dopamine D2 receptors), familial development and the problem of chromosome 5 have not been settled. In the future, when all symptoms can be explained materially, psychiatry will be largely integrated into neurology. However, even then, the question of "What is the spiritual matter?" from the functional aspect of psychiatry will likely remain, but the current situation is far from being resolved.

In terms of brain function, schizophrenia seems to be caused by (reversible, partial) enhancement, and dementia, on the contrary, by (chronic) decline. However, the opposite (negative symptoms in schizophrenia, agitation in dementia) can also occur. For diagnosis and treatment, even that level of recognition is not insufficient at present (that level of awareness is permissible).

Can schizophrenia and dementia be differentiated to some extent by imaging test?

Geriatric-onset LOS and VLOS have some imaging features (though not as definitive features as dementia). Cerebrovascular lesions in the fronto-tempo-parietal lobe of the right hemisphere (the location is not well defined, but it is often on the right side), organic changes in the temporal lobe and orbital surface of the frontal lobe are related to the neural and organic basis of hallucinations and delusions.

It is difficult to distinguish schizophrenia and dementia from other images, and there is no choice but to distinguish from symptoms and progress. That is, in dementia, argyrophilic grain dementia among FTLD, DLB, and AD tend to cause symptoms similar to those of schizophrenia in that order, and it is difficult to distinguish between schizophrenia and dementia. However, in FTLD, the organic disorder progresses when the progress is observed. By the way, deep white matter lesions are prone to depressive symptoms. Auditory and visual hallucinations are much more frequent in DLB than in AD. Delusions are often associated with phantom housemates. When visual hallucinations and auditory hallucinations are combined, it becomes intractable.

§8 Memory disturbance in dementia

What is the mechanism of memory in the first place? Papez circuit is a main important circuit of memory centered on the hippocampus. Most of the parts of the brain that cause amnesia are Papez circuits: hippocampus → cerebral fornix → mammary body → anterior thalamic nucleus → cingulate gyrus → hippocampus. It is mainly related to short-term episodic memory (For instance, I went to Koshien Stadium to watch the Hanshin Tigers' game yesterday), and Korsakoff's syndrome (recent memory impairment, confabulation, disorientation) is famous for disorders of this circuit.

Yakovlev circuit is emotions related neural networks centered on the amygdala. Memories related to emotions such as happiness, joy, and sadness are well remembered even in the past: amygdala → dorsomedial thalamus → anterior cingulate gyrus → posterior orbital cortex of frontal lobe → anterior temporal lobe → amygdala.

The hippocampus and the amygdala are adjacent sites that are closely related to each other. The Yakovlev and Papez circuits interact and cooperate to perform efficient actions.

Remote memory consists of three processes: memorization (encoding), retention (storage), and recall (retrieval). After processing and encoding information, we memorize it, and "retain" what I have remembered. The more clues to search for memory are memorized together, the easier it is to remember (you can associate and recall from the many keywords). We create new neural circuits, and this is the process for transferring short-term memory to long-term memory. The function of recalling long-term memory is retrieval with "recall". Retrievals of the memory are further divided into two. "Recollection (retrieval)" includes "reproduction" (to reproduce the retained memory in its original form and recall it freely) and "recognition" (selective recall of previously remembered events and experiences). It can be divided into two types: A baby cries when it is comforted by a stranger because it recognizes (that is, recognizes) the difference between the face of its mother, who is always there for it and treats it kindly, and the face of its mother who is not. This is recognition memory, the representative of which is shyness. There is also reconstruction (the process of combining and reproducing some of the retained memories).

Pathway between cerebral cortex and hippocampus are related to the remote memory of "I came first in the relay at the elementary school athletic meet." First, recent memories formed in the hippocampus are temporarily

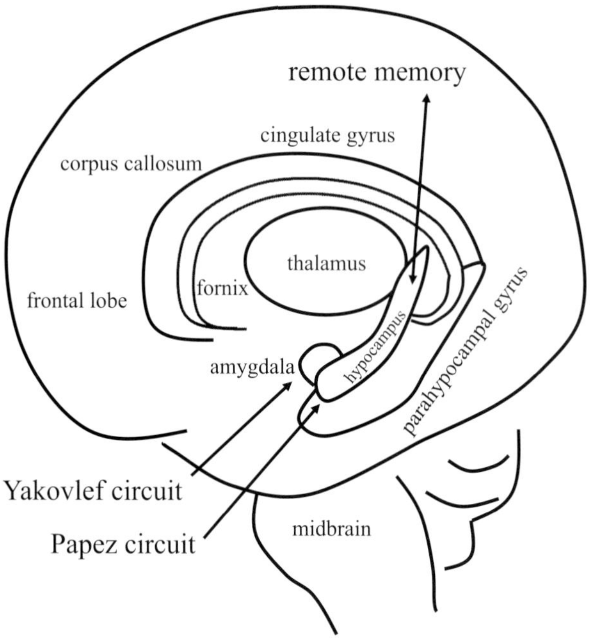

Fig.6. Simple schema for understanding memory circuits.

stored in the hippocampus and then transferred to the cerebral cortex (Fig.6).

People with dementia remember things from the past well, but forget new things. Why is this? Rather than forgetting new things, Papez's circuit (around the hippocampus) and others were malfunctioning due to AD, and the main cause was that the patient could not remember accurately in the recent phase. He can remember what he memorized correctly. The areas in charge of recent memory and old memory are different. Remote memory (becoming first in the relay at the elementary school athletic meet) is related to the cerebral cortex and hippocampus. First, recent memories formed in the hippocampus are temporarily stored in the hippocampus and then transferred to the cerebral cortex for storage. When recalling memories, memory traces left in the hippocampus act on the cerebral cortex to recall memories (Makino Y, et al : Cell Reports 10:1016, 2019).

§9 Choline hypothesis

Acetylcholine (Ach) is the most markedly decreased neurotransmitter in AD brain, and cholinergic nerve disorder has been analyzed in detail. In the 1970s and 1980s, it was reported that disorders of cholinergic nerves were deeply related to memory and cognitive ability, and the choline hypothesis was postulated. In fact, abnormalities in the cholinergic nervous system are remarkable in AD brains. That is, degeneration and disappearance of cholinergic neurons that project "from the basal nucleus of Meynert in the basal forebrain to the cerebral cortex," and "from the septal nucleus and nucleus of the diagonal band of Broca to the hippocampal body." This phenomenon occurs, and as a result, the input to the cerebral cortex and hippocampus is severely impaired, resulting in a decrease in the amount of Ach.

Ach esterase (Ache) inhibitors, including donepezil, have been developed for the purpose of replenishing the decreased Ach and alleviating the symptoms of dementia. According to the theory, when Ache inhibitors increase the amount of Ach that binds to post-synaptic membrane receptors and improve the efficiency of neurotransmission, cholinergic input is activated and cognitive impairment is alleviated. It is a drug treatment for the core symptom. The core symptom is mainly memory impairment, and antidementia drugs (four types: donepezil, galantamine, rivastigmine, and memantine) are often tried, but they are not very effective (at our hospital, about 20% of dementia patients were medicated).

In France, antidementia drugs have been removed from insurance coverage. Four drugs have been excluded from medical insurance coverage in France since August 2018. The French Ministry of Solidarity and Health announced that it had evaluated its effectiveness 7 years earlier as low, but in 2016 it further evaluated it as inadequate, leading to this decision. The authorities judged that the efficacy of the drug was not high considering the side effects, and that the usefulness of the drug was insufficient. The patients paid the full amount themselves.

Theoretically, memory impairment, which is the most important core symptom, should be a local symptom caused by an organic lesion caused by a disorder of the Papez or Yakovlev's circuit, but we have necessarily not found an organic lesion in these circuits. Moreover, it is not always the case that a local organic causative focus that is thought to be symptomatically consistent with peripheral symptoms is recognized.

In Japan, there were many opinions that it was effective in improving cognitive function. There is still no movement to remove it from insurance coverage in Japan, but the effect is limited. There are quite a few voices pointing out that. In Japan, 17% of the elderly received prescriptions for antidementia drugs (2015).

§10 Mechanism of BPSD

BPSD is said to be related to neurotransmitters rather than symptoms caused by local organic abnormalities. In addition, depression occurs by the following mechanism (again, it is not caused by organic abnormalities), and the balanced relationship between serotonin, dopamine, and adrenaline mainly controls the mental state ("monoamine hypothesis") (Healy D: Psychopharmacol 11(4 suppl), S25,1997).

That is, when the serotonin system is dysfunctional, aggression increases, anxiety, fear, and panic. Noradrenergic hyperfunction causes restlessness, increased aggression, and irritability. Behavioral abnormalities and increased aggression is due to hyperfunction of the dopamine system. In addition, due to Ach system dysfunction, hyperactivity, increased aggression, psychiatric symptoms, etc. have been reported so far. Although there is a strong desire among medical practitioners to treat the appearance of BPSD as a localized symptom of the brain, it is somewhat difficult.

Now, what should be the drug treatment for BPSD? Drug therapy is not performed from the beginning. However, if the positive symptoms are urgent or too pronounced, drug therapy should be considered.

Among antipsychotics, atypical antipsychotics should be used if medication is to be used (there are fewer side effects such as EPS than typical antipsychotics). Since the typical type of antipsychotics blocks all dopaminergic nervous systems, EPS is likely to occur (chlorpromazine, haloperidol, and tiapride are typical examples). The atypical type primarily blocks the mesolimbic dopamine pathway, but less the nigrostriatal dopamine pathway (typically risperidone, quetiapine, aripiprazole). Antidementia drugs may be effective against BPSD (e.g., donepezil for hallucinations, delusions, and apathy in dementia with Lewy bodies. Galantamine for hallucinations and sleep disturbances).

Treatment of dementia

§11 Psychotropics and antipsychotics

Classification of psychotropic drugs

1. antipsychotics
   Typical antipsychotics : haloperidol, chlorpromazine
   Atypical antipsychotics
   Serotonin dopamine antagonist (SDA): risperidone
   MARTA: quetiapine, olanzapine
   Dopamine D2 partial agonist (DPA): aripiprazole
2. antidepressants
   Selective serotonin reuptake inhibitor (SSRI): paroxetine (Paxil)
   Serotonin noradrenaline reuptake inhibitor (SNRI): duloxetine (Cymbalta)
   NaSSA: mirtazapine
   TCA tricyclic drug: Tryptanol
3. mood stabilizer: lithium carbonate (Limas)
4. psychostimulants: methamphetamine

What are antipsychotics?

Antipsychotics is one of psychotropic drugs and a general term for drugs that are a type of drugs that have antipsychotic effects. They are used for schizophrenia, schizoaffective disorder, delusional disorder, bipolar disorder, severe depressive state, problem behavior of dementia (violence, excitement), hallucinatory delusions, artificial experiences (others try to manipulate the patient into doing something), psychomotor agitation, intense anxiety, irritability, and other psychotic symptoms and psychiatric disorders. It is classified as follows according to the development age.

The 1st generation: Typical antipsychotics such as phenothiazine derivatives, used less frequently these days, but traditionally highly favored by psychiatrists. Phenothiazine type chlorpromazine, Hirunamine, Wintamine (they have strong sedative effect), amitriptyline (Tryptanol). Butyrophenone-type haloperidol (Serenase) (they have effects on hallucinations and delusions). Benzamide-type sulpiride (Dogmatyl), tiapride (Gramalil) (they tend to cause EPS). In general, they tend to cause adverse effect such as orthostatic hypotension, Parkinson symptom, malignant symptom, tardive dyskinesia. So then I don't use these drugs much.

The 2nd generation: Atypical antipsychotics, which tend to have fewer side effects than typical antipsychotics. Zolpidem, risperidone, olanzapine, quetiapine, paroxetine, clozapine, blonanserin, etc.

The 3rd generation: It has a stabilizing effect on dopamine transmission through a mechanism different from that of the 1st and 2nd generation. Aripiprazole and others fall into this category.

Aripiprazole, risperidone

They are frequently used in antipsychotics. Aripiprazole is DPA. It antagonizes the increased dopamine D2 receptors in the mesolimbic system and moderately activates the other decreased dopamine D2 receptors. That is, they are partial agonists. It has less EPS. It has an antagonistic effect on the 5-HT2 receptor of serotonin, a partial stimulatory effect on the 5-HT1 receptor, and an ameliorating effect on the negative symptoms of BPSD evoked by serotonin.

Risperidone is SDA. Dopamine and serotonin have an antagonistic relationship, but the serotonin-blocking action is stronger. It suppresses positive symptoms by blocking dopamine in the mesolimbic system. Negative symptoms occur in the mesocortical system due to lack of dopamine. Since SDA blocks 5-HT2A receptors, dopamine, which had been suppressed by serotonin in the mesocortical system, is released, improving negative symptoms. D2 receptor blockade reduces nigrostriatal dopamine function and causes EPS. In order that blockage of 5-HT2A receptor does not weaken dopamine action too much, it is expected that EPS will be less likely to occur. Since the action of dopamine on the hypothalamus is maintained, the side effects of increased prolactin are slightly lessened. There are side effects such as body weight gain, lipid and blood sugar increase, orthostatic hypotension, and QT prolongation.

Concerning the side effects of antipsychotic drugs, as for that of typical antipsychotics, symptoms of EPS (acute dystonia such as sursumversion, involuntary movements of the neck, limbs, and trunk, and muscle stiffness), malignant syndrome, orthostatic hypotension, and hypothalamic-pituitary system disorders are prominently observed to compare with those of the atypical one.

§12 Polypharmacy issue

Most of psychotropic drugs are metabolized by cytochrome P450 (CYP). That's where the problem of polypharmacy comes in. In conclusion, polypharmacy must be inhibited because we may further additionally administer psychotropic drugs after hospitalization. Polypharmacy is considered to be drug-induced frailty. Most antipsychotic drugs are metabolized by CYP. When a dementia patient is transferred to a convalescent rehabilitation hospital, we ask the family, the patient, or the key person to consider whether they will allow to change or reduce their medication. It is necessary to consider the possibility of administering additional antipsychotic drugs after admission, and to correct polypharmacy itself other than psychotropic drugs from the time of admission. In addition to correction, it is also important to know the way of thinking of family members or key persons. One week after hospitalization is necessary to improve relocation damage, that is, to improve the environment, get used to the new environment and stabilize or understand the general condition. In parallel with them we improve polypharmacy. It is then that a new medication is started if necessary.

It is not uncommon for patients to be prescribed more than 10 types of medication when they are admitted to a convalescent hospital after visiting multiple general practitioners, primary care physicians, and acute care hospitals.

Drugs (mostly fat-soluble) are absorbed from the small intestine (Absorption). Only the free form that is not bound to albumin is distributed to the tissue cells of the target organ (Distribution) and exerts a medicinal effect. During several cycles through the liver, fat-soluble drugs are metabolized to water-soluble by CYP in the microsome of the endoplasmic reticulum of the liver (Metabolism) and excreted by the kidneys or bile (Excretion). The four steps are the principl of the pharmacokinetics.

The "first-pass effect" means that the drug is absorbed from the small intestine, metabolized in the liver via the portal vein, and enters the systemic circulatory system, but at the time when the drug first passes through the liver and is metabolized, the drug is inactivated to some extent and the action is attenuated. As the drug passes through the systemic circulation and constantly passes through the liver, it is metabolized, deactivated and become water-soluble, and finally completely excreted by the kidneys.

The first step in the transition of the drug into the brain is that the drug is fat-soluble and has a low molecular weight, which allows it to cross the blood-brain barrier. Some water-soluble drugs can be passed through active transport using Mt.

CYP is an oxidase consisting of 500 amino acid residues. CYP is an enzyme that detoxifies in the liver, and is present in the endoplasmic reticulum and some Mt in cells. The fat-soluble drugs became water-soluble and are excreted from the kidneys as mentioned above.

Metabolism of the drug is carried out through two stages: phase I (oxidation, reduction, hydrolysis) and phase II (conjugation reaction).

In the first phase, CYP undergoes an oxidation reaction (catalyzed by CYP-based drug-metabolizing enzymes) to improve water solubility and finally facilitate excretion from the body. The second phase (the conjugation reaction) is a reaction in which a substance with high water solubility material (such as glucuronic acid) binds to the drug to increase the water solubility and facilitate excretion.

There are 60 molecular species of CYP, but only a few of them are important in clinical practice (involved in 80~90% of all drug metabolism). Since all antipsychotics, except paliperidone (it is a metabolite of risperidone and excreted by the kidneys), are metabolized by CYPs in the liver, great care must be taken regarding possible polypharmacy disorders. However, the relationship between the enzyme name and the drug is very complicated and difficult to remember. Therefore, healthcare professionals should be aware of the interaction and pharmacokinetic items in the attached documents if there is any problem in administering the drug to the patient. When discussing metabolism by CYPs, it is important to consider drug interactions, which include competition (decrease drug action), inhibitory effects (increase drug action) and metabolic induction (decrease drug action).

In discussing drug interactions, the basic academic terms for elements which becomes the basis of the metabolism of drugs are "substrates" (they are drugs originally administered, and the effects are affected in various ways), "inhibitors" (other drugs which may inhibit and slow the metabolism of substrates, thereby increasing blood levels). The third basic elements are "drug inducers" (other drugs that increase metabolic enzymes and accelerate drug metabolism, making the drug less effective). Metabolic induction occurs due to activation of transcription in cells.

There are three types of inhibition of CYP: competitive inhibition, non-specific inhibition, and irreversible inhibition.

Nonspecific inhibition reversibly inhibits multiple CYP molecular species by coordinating binding to heme iron at the active center of CYP. Cimetidine and azole antifungal drugs are typical and well-known. Non-specifically inhibits multiple CYP molecular species in a non-selective manner. In particular, strong inhibition of CYP2D6 and CYP3A4 was observed. The concentration of the inhibited drug in the blood becomes too high, which is dangerous. In fact, cimetidine strongly inhibits CYP2D6, and azole antifungals strongly inhibit

CYP3A4.

Competitive inhibition occurs when multiple substrates are metabolized in a single CYP, inhibiting drugs with low affinity and increasing their blood levels, but not changing blood concentrations of drugs with high affinity.

When a drug is metabolized by CYP, irreversible inhibition may occur. Metabolites generated by the catalytic action of CYP react irreversibly with CYP (binding to heme and apoproteins) to form a complex and the inhibitory action continues indefinitely. This phenomenon is called "mechanism based inhibition (MBI)." Even after the inhibitor disappears from the body, a persistent inhibitory effect is observed, and serious side effects appear. Erythromycin, spironolactone, grapefruit and others can cause irreversible inhibition (Yoshinari K:Folia Pharmacol Jpn.134:285, 2009) .

If we say very roughly about the drugs that are commonly used in the area of convalescent rehabilitation, medications to be aware of include:

CYP1A2: substrates are olanzapine (MARTA) and ramelteon. The inducer is omeprazole and smoking (drug efficacy is reduced). Metabolism is induced by smoking (smoking reduces efficacy).

CYP2C9: Substrates are warfarin and diclofenac.

CYP2C19: Substrates are omeprazole, lansoprazole, clopidogrel and diazepam. Clopidogrel is a prodrug and is activated when metabolized by CYP2C19. Conversely, lansoprazole loses activity when metabolized by CYP2C19. Therefore, clopidogrel was ineffective in patients who responded to lansoprazole. What is important in CYP2C19 is the existence of genetic polymorphism. 20% of Japanese are poor metabolizers and do not have much CYP2C19 activity (hypometabolic forms). Clopidogrel is a prodrug and is activated by being metabolized in CYP2C19. Poor metabolizer has little enzyme activity, so clopidogrel is almost ineffective. Conversely, lansoprazole, which loses its activity by being metabolized in the CYP2C19, is strongly effective in poor metabolizers.

CYP2D6: More than 25% of drugs are metabolized by this. The substrates are Tryptanol, aripiprazole and risperidone. The inhibitor is paroxetine, and the inducer is dexamethasone. Genetic polymorphisms are also present in CYP2D6 (1% of Japanese are poor metabolizer), but intermediate metabolizers are said to be relatively abundant (slightly lower metabolitive).

CYP2E1: Substrate is acetaminophen, inducer is ethanol (drinking).

CYP3A4: Substrates are warfarin, nifedipine, Xarelto, perospirone, aripiprazole, quetiapine and diltiazem. The inducer is dexamethasone. The inhibitor is grapefruit. Other CYPs are present only in the liver, while CYP3A4 is present in the liver and small intestine. It is involved in the metabolism of more than 50% of medicines.

§13 Non-pharmacological treatment for BPSD

Non-pharmacological treatment should be given for BPSD first. The treatment is psychotherapy. The person-centered care proposed by Thomas Marris Kitwood of UK (1937-1998, pastor and psychotherapist) is a treatment method that respects the individuality of the patient from the perspective and standpoint of the patient. Then further, a new method called Humanitude has been developed by Yves Gineste and Rosette Marescotti of France (both were physical education teachers) since 1979. It is a care technique that improves the relationship with people complicated by dementia and enables smooth communication. Furthermore, validation therapy is founded by Naomi Feil of US. For details of these psychotherapies, please refer to other written books or the Internet.

§14 Factors that promote exacerbation of dementia

Pharmacological and non-pharmacological treatments for dementia are mainly symptomatic treatments for BPSD except for D2 abnormality. In the meantime, the pathological stage of dementia (brain changes) is progressing. It is important to proceed with aggressive treatment for dementia exacerbation factors (pathology) in parallel. What are the exacerbation factors?

1. DM

Exacerbation promoting factors include hyperglycemia (AGE-RAGE), hypoglycemia (endoplasmic reticulum stress), and diurnal variation in blood glucose levels. Although their mechanisms are different, they ultimately cause neuronal damage due to oxidative stress. Furthermore, in DM, a decrease in insulin degrading enzyme, which disassembles amyloidβ, is a factor that promotes exacerbation, and as a result, the degradation of amyloidβ in brain tissue is decreased, so amyloid accumulates in the brain (normally, insulin degrading enzyme decomposes amyloid in brain tissue, leading to escape from dementia).

In addition, impaired arteriolar circulation due to DM also adversely affects dementia. Glucose uptake into nerve cells is reduced, insulin resistance of nerve cells is increased, the effect of insulin is reduced, and nerve cell damage progresses. In short, when AD patients have DM, AD progresses faster.

2. Sleep disturbance

Amyloid β is decomposed during sleep, but decomposition is suppressed in sleep disorders.

3. Severe illness causing SIRS, CARS, etc.

HMGB-1, which is the necrotic substance of the causative disease, binds to RAGE, and CARS persists, AGEs-RAGE increases, neuronal damage persists, and dementia progresses. IL6 may be measured as an indicator of CARS. The elderly patients with severe illness sometimes develops dementia during hospitalization. Patients admitted to convalescent rehabilitation often have 1-3, mentioned above.

Alzheimer's disease

§15 Characteristics and overview of AD

AD accounts for more than 50% of all dementia cases and is slightly more common in women. Cognitive impairment gradually progresses mainly in middle-aged and older people. Since the medial temporal lobe, which is related to memory, and the Meynert nucleus, which is related to the metabolism of Ach, are impaired, it begins with memory impairment (first, recent episode memory impairment). In the dementia test, memory of the word cannot be kept 5 minutes, and cannot recollect. Symptoms begin with core symptoms (mainly memory impairment), and peripheral symptoms also appear as the disease progresses. Movement disorders are not recognized until late in the disease (it presents at the end).

Histopathologically, harmful amyloid β (produced by not only the patients but also anyone) accumulates in the brain. Amyloid β gradually accumulates outside nerve cells and forms small masses called senile plaques due to a decline in the function of microglia, which has the function of removing this. In succession, neurofibrillary tangles occur in nerve cells, leading to degeneration and necrosis of nerve cells. That is, neuropathologically, the following two major findings appear (Braak H, et al: Acta Neuropathol 82: 239, 1991).

1. senile plaque

It is composed of amyloid β protein outside nerve cells (aggregate accumulation). Senile plaques develop in the order of neocortex → hippocampus → primary cortex (Braak's senile plaque stage classification). PET examination enables early detection of the distribution of amyloid-β deposits in the brain.

2. neurofibrillary tangles

Neurofibrillary tangles composed of phosphorylated tau protein (one of the microtubule-associated proteins) in neurons. It progresses in the order of trans-entorhinal cortex→ limbal system → neocortex), and degeneration of neurons disappears, causing cerebral atrophy (Braak's stage classification of neurofibrillary tangles). The order of progression of neurofibrillary tangle is different from that of senile plaque.

For the above pathological findings, it is necessary to collect specimens by biopsy or autopsy of the patient's brain, which is impossible in daily clinical practice, but those who are interested can easily observe the pathological findings on the Internet. PET examination enables early detection of the distribution of amyloid β deposits in the brain, but this is not covered by health insurance and is not used for general AD diagnosis. Academically, researcher are very interested. Anyone can see this on the Internet. None of the AD inpatients in the convalescent ward of our hospital underwent PET.

AD is classified into early-onset type and late-onset type. Early onset type is under age 65: familial AD with autosomal dominant inheritance (Ages 18-39 : Early-onset dementia. Ages 40-64 : Presenile dementia).

Late-onset type (after age 65): This is the majority of AD. No family history (i.e., sporadic). Associated gene (risk factor that promotes onset) is apolipoprotein E4 allele gene polymorphism on chromosome 19 (10% of Japanese people have). It is more likely to occur 4 times more than those who do not have the gene and the age of onset is lower.

Early-onset AD and late-onset AD differs in the progression of brain atrophy. Early-onset AD (aged 65 or younger) with rapid progression of cognitive decline such as marked apraxia and agnosia. Hippocampal atrophy is not conspicuous, while late-onset AD is characterized by hippocampal atrophy.

Concerning diagnosis of AD, in accordance with AD diagnosis guidelines of the NIA-AA, the presence of dementia, slow progression from several months to more than a year, and we meet more than one of the impairment in the areas among amnesia, aphasia, visuospatial function, and executive function (McKhann GM, et al : Alzheimer's Dement 7:263,2011). There are many people with dementia that meet this relatively lax criteria, and it is difficult to diagnose AD just by meeting this guideline (details about the case report described later).

Sporadic AD

In sporadic AD, environmental factors other than genes (related genes mentioned below) are related to the onset. Adverse effects on risk of onset include: ageing (greatest risk is ageing), family history of AD, Down syndrome, late child bearing, cerebrovascular disease, hypertension, smoking, obesity, head injury, high blood pressure, hypercholesterolemia, diabetes (1.3～1.8-fold in diabetic patients, 2-fold with insulin injections), and 5.5-fold with the ApoEε4 allele on chromosome 19. Conversely, the factors that reduce the risk of onset are: lifestyle, education (intellectual lifestyle), leisure activities, exercise habits, diet (Mediterranean diet such as Italian, Spanish, Greek, etc. containing olive oil), various food (blue-backed fish, green tea and red wine polyphenols, flavonoids containing antioxidants along with polyphenols, fruits and vegetables, beta-carotene, high intake of antioxidants such as vitamin C, vitamin E), and drugs (estrogen, calcium channel blockers, NSAIDs, although none of these can be used regularly due to side effects).

Familial AD

Concerning causative and related genes of familial AD, there are multiple causative genes: three causative genes and one related gene have been identified.

The causative gene is the amyloid precursor protein (APP) gene on chromosome 21, the presenilin 1 gene on chromosome 14, and the presenilin 2 gene on chromosome 1.

The related gene is the apolipoprotein E4 gene on chromosome 19, which is carried by 10% of Japanese. People with abnormality of the apolipoprotein E4 gene are 4 times more likely to develop AD than people without it.

Incidence of familial AD is 1% of all AD, usually inherited in an autosomal dominant manner. Some take the form of recessive inheritance. Even if there are no abnormalities in the above-mentioned causative genes or related genes, it is said that the risk of AD is slightly increased if there is a relative with AD. In particular, if there is a relative who developed the disease at the age of 50-54, the risk of early onset of the disease is about 20 times higher.

§16 Symptoms and clinical course of AD

AD is characterized by slow onset and persistent cognitive decline, and MMSE decreases by an average of 3-4 points per year. In general, the younger the patient, the faster the onset and progression. As the course progresses, myoclonus and convulsions are seen in about 10%. In the final stage, the patient becomes bedridden with aphasia. It is said that it takes 5±3 years from the onset until about half of the patients become bedridden, and the mean duration of illness until death is 8 to 12 years.

Symptoms that are more characteristic of AD than other dementias are:

Early stage: Characterized by word recall disorder, visuospatial cognitive disorder, temporal disorientation (others include recent memory disorder, episodic memory disorder, compositional apraxia, word finding difficulty).

Middle stage: Characterized by place disorientation, ideological apraxia (impaired use of objects, e.g. inability to use an electric shaver). Others are route disorder, topographical memory disorder.

Complementing the characteristic symptoms of AD:

Among the disorientation disorders, they are impaired

in the order of time, place, and person. The initial symptoms noticed by family members are memory impairment: forgetting quickly, hearing and saying the same thing over and over again, forgetting to misplace or misplace, forgetting names of people, things, writing in Chinese characters, turning on water and fire, taking medicine, and forgetting route, place related to disorientation. Loss of previous interest or lack of routine, or sloppiness. Persecutory paranoia such as irritability, skeptical personality changes, having his wallet stolen, or being abused by family members. Increased mistakes in work or housework, calculation errors, comprehension ability such as inability to understand the content of complicated TV dramas, other disorders of executive function, attention disorders, etc. When asked about something he doesn't understand, he doesn't answer "I don't know" and make some kind of excuse. For example, when asked what kind of food he is good at, he doesn't give specific names of food, such as "I can make anything" or "It is ordinary", but he tries to cover it up so as not to make it look like a mess. It is also common to look back at the spouse beside him and ask for help. In moderate AD, immediate memory impairment (remembering a few seconds ago), distant memory impairment from the closest order, and vocabulary decrease also progressed. In severe AD, almost all memories are impaired, and the disorientation of time and place progresses further, making it impossible to distinguish between morning and afternoon, and to judge whether it is home or not. Others: From 2 to 10 years later, the personality becomes a mere skeleton losing substance: he greet people on the street and speak politely with relatives at events such as memorial services. Greetings such as "It's nice weather today", "Thanks to you, I'm fine", and the art of ad hoc conversation learned over many years are not easily lost (honorifics and polite manners). By the way, what is meant by "metamorphosis" is that the rules and mechanisms do not function and become only a form. As a side note, "form" means the body (without the soul). During this period, behavioral problems such as wandering and unclean behavior also appears.

§17 Aphasia associated with AD

Conversation with only pronouns such as "that, that" for anonymity, word amnesia and repetition of irrelevant topics are also characteristical. Speech fluency is initially preserved, and repetition is relatively good, but auditory comprehension impairment, reading and writing impairment (more pronounced in kanji than in kana) are observed. Conversation without content occurs due to reduced vocabulary and spontaneous speech. As it progresses, parroting the other person's words (echolinguistic echolalia) and repeating the same words (cologous repetition, palilalia). Ultimately, they become silent and unable to understand what we say, and are indifferent and uninterested.

§18 Bizarre symptoms of dementia

These are not necessarily characteristic of AD but there is a bizarre syndrome that is a little different from BPSD. They are common in dementia or other psychiatric disorders such as schizophrenia.

Charles Bonnet syndrome: Long-term deprivation of visual stimuli in elderly people with visual system disorders leads to hyperactivity of the cerebral cortex, resulting in DLB-like visual hallucinations.

Capgras syndrome: Someone impersonates person close to you, such as your wife. The most in schizophrenia. It is also common in AD and DLB.

Othello syndrome: Delusions that the spouse is unfaithful (related to delusions that the spouse may abandon the patient).

Cotard's syndrome: Hypochondriacal delusions that some organs are rotting (immortal delusions; I cannot die anymore).

Fregoli's illusion: The man (unknown) sitting next to the patient is her husband in disguise.

Clerambault syndrome: Delusional illusion of being loved (loved delusion).

Diogenes syndrome: Isolated elderly people become careless about their appearance, accumulating unnecessary things and turning into garbage houses.

Pareidolia test: Mistaking nonsensical figures for faces. Due to visuospatial cognitive impairment, configuration disorder. Marked in posterior cortical atrophy, common in AD, and common in also DLB. Besides, delusional misperceptions are also common in DLB, often accompanied by visual hallucinations.

Phantom cohabitant: Someone patient doesn't know is living in the house, such as in the attic, and doing bad things (torturing the patient). A lot in schizophrenia.

Mirror phenomenon: The patient sees a stranger in the mirror (despite the reflection of the patient himself in the mirror).

Godot syndrome: Asking about future events or appointments over and over again. When it gets worse, it is a burden for caregivers.

Metamorphopsia: The shape and size of an object change while looking at it.

Just illusions : Just illusions are many. People, small animals, insects, children, etc.

Music box clock symptom: Timetable living with stereotyped behaviors at fixed times each day. Seen in FTLD.

Optical illusion: Curtains and hanging clothes appear to be a man.

§19 Apraxia associated with dementia

1. Constructive disability and symptoms of dementia, such as difficulty in drawing and copying clocks and three-dimensional figures are observed (Fig.7).
2. Ideational apraxia (use disorder of daily necessities and articles), ideomotor apraxia (imitation disorder, pantomime disorder of simple movements), and limb-kinetic apraxia, etc. are observed.
3. Dressing apraxia (inability to choose appropriate clothes, inability to put on clothes, etc.) progresses in conjunction with deficits in procedural memory (how to ride a bicycle, etc.). He can't do self-care eventually such as grooming, dressing, eating, toileting, and bathing.
4. In the terminal stage, it progresses to the loss of basic motor skills such as standing, sitting, and walking.

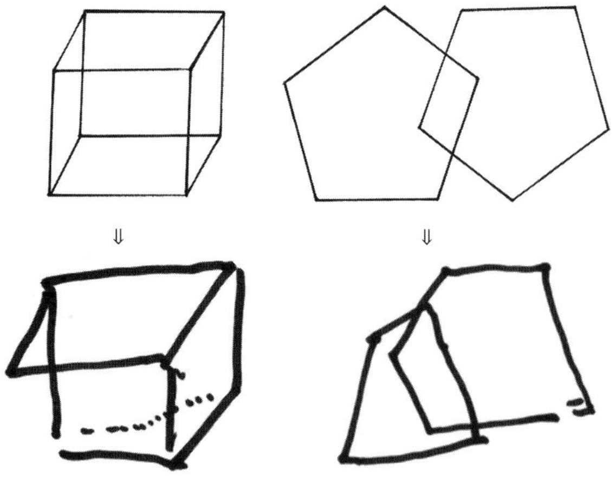

Fig.7. Examination of constructive disability and symptoms of dementia showing difficulty in drawing and copying three-dimensional figures.

Agnosia associated with dementia, especially AD

1. In the early stages, patients have a visual spatial perception disorder, a disorder of visual calculation, visual estimation of the positional relationship with size, and perspective of objects. He is not good at backing up a car in the garage.
2. In the middle stage, disorientation to places is observed, namely route disorder and topographical memory disorder, which causes wandering.
3. As the disease progresses, it becomes impossible to identify family members due to prosopagnosia and person misidentification. Capgras syndrome, phantom housemates, mirror phenomenon, etc.

BPSD associated with AD

1. Delusions of persecution, being hidden or being stolen, and delusions of jealousy are observed.
2. Personality changes such as sharpening of pre-morbid personality and lack of methodicalness, slovenly grooming, and tidying up the room appears.
3. In the middle stage, the patient loses insight into the disease, becomes euphoric, and progresses to apathy and indifference.
4. In moderate to severe AD, changes in eating behavior, overeating, social deviant behavior, sexual disinhibition, clinging, repeating the same question, increased dependence, twilight syndrome that says to go home at dusk, setting his eyes, wandering around going out and getting lost, collection habit that fills the room with trivial things, sleep-wake rhythm disorder, resistance to nursing care, etc. appear.
5. In severe AD, positive symptoms such as walking around inside and outside the house, loitering outside, shouting loudly at night, screaming, playing with defecation, violence, verbal abuse, and vandalism appear. At the same time as nursing care becomes difficult in his

home, it becomes unmanageable for family doctors.

§20 Illustrative case of typical AD

§15 described the lax diagnostic criteria for AD, and I explain why the diagnostic criteria are lax in this section. I present a case to help you understand that the diagnosis of AD cannot be confirmed by diagnostic criteria alone. I want you to understand the reason from the contents of my following case report of 87-year-old female presenting with recent memory impairment and nocturnal delirium. This case report is interspersed with characteristic medical histories, symptoms, and signs suggestive of AD, suggesting that it is impossible to consider cases other than AD.

[Life history] This 87-year-old female graduated from an elementary school in a village in the countryside, depth of the mountains of the Chugoku region, and got married to a man in the same village. Her diet consists mainly of wild vegetables in Japanese cuisine (as a matter of course, he does not eat Mediterranean cuisine). She often eats fruits (which contain vitamin C) (mandarin oranges, etc.). No drinking or smoking. She doesn't like print and doesn't watch TV or read newspapers. After living a peaceful life in a farming village, she moved to his son's neighborhood X-10 years ago.

[Family history] She has one son (no dementia).

[History of current illness]

X-5 years ago recent memory impairment and wandering have appeared. She suffered from pelvic fracture while wandering. She consulted a psychiatrist and was diagnosed with AD, and started oral treatment with antidementia drugs. Her husband provided care for her, and conversely she cared for him.

X-4 years she was separated by her husband' death and has lived alone. Since then, she has stopped doing housework due to executive dysfunction, and has become neglectful in maintaining her house (garbage house) and socializing with neighbors. Her son and his wife living near the patient started taking care of her, but it is difficult for the patient to live alone.

X-3 year ago she entered facility. Occasionally she came back to her house or her son's house, but she had a habit of collecting (getting a lot of toilet paper from the facility), a delusion of things being stolen (she suspected that her pen would be taken by his son's wife), and recent episodic memory impairment, paranoia, self-centeredness and aggressiveness, nocturnal delirium, day-night reversal, etc. were conspicuous.

On X-20 day, she fell out of bed while in a facility and underwent osteosynthesis at a hospital for her left femoral trochanteric fracture. She transferred to our hospital on X-day for rehabilitation.

[Current condition]

Neurologically: Her core symptoms are recent and episodic memory impairment. Her memory is fuzzy, and her son's wife corrects her wrong remarks when she is not around.

Her BPSD is:

1. Twilight syndrome (anxiety is noticeable before dinner)
2. Nocturnal delirium
3. She has persecution delusions (frequently calling staff and making irrelevant requests. Some remarks, "Why don't you care more? I'm the only one being discriminated."). She has reversal of day and night, and these symptoms continue until midnight.
4. Cognitive dysfunction: In addition to prehospital executive dysfunction (described above), she requires assistance due to clothing apraxia (wearing the jacket inside out). Because of geographical disorder, she cannot go back from the hospital cafeteria or toilet and sleep in someone else's bed. As a language disorder, she does not like printing from the beginning, has anonymity and has decreased vocabulary, and has increased pronouns.

[Laboratory findings]

1. HDS-R 11/30, MMSE 14/30 (disorientation, short-term memory impairment, delayed recall task impairment).
2. MRI: Bilateral medial temporal lobe atrophy and hippocampal atrophy are prominent. There is no atrophy of the midbrain tegmentum, innominate substance and hypothalamus (Fig.8) . Atrophy of the cerebral cortex is age-appropriate.

[Basis leading to the diagnosis of AD]

1. Consistent with dementia according to the DSM-5 diagnostic criteria for cognitive impairment (2013).
2. MRI findings are consistent with AD.
3. Differential diagnosis includes Creutzfeldt-Jakob disease, frontotemporal lobar degeneration, dementia with

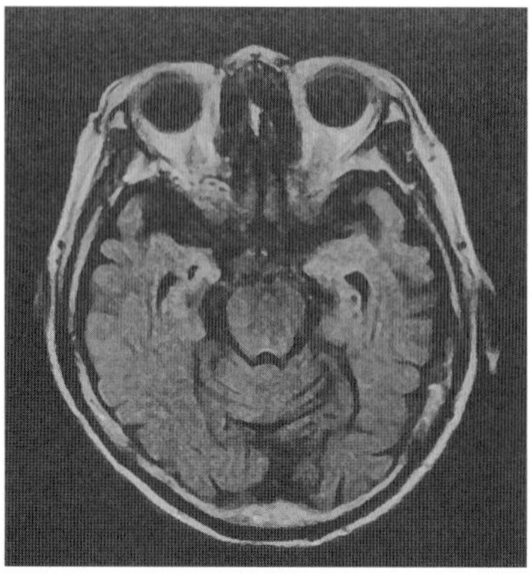

Fig.8. MRI: Bilateral medial temporal lobe atrophy and hippocampal atrophy are prominent, which is compatible with AD. There is no other lesion in the brain.

Lewy bodies, dementia due to other neurodegenerative diseases, vascular dementia, etc. There are no suspicious clinical symptoms, laboratory findings, or their clinical courses that make the above diseases suspected.

4. It meets diagnostic criteria for AD (2011). There is no dementia in the family history, and for several years (from the age of 82) deterioration of cognitive function, progression of amnesia, appearance of aphasia, and decline in executive function were observed. Other dementia diseases were negated from MRI findings and symptoms. Consequently, I make diagnosis of sporadic late-onset AD showing FAST 5.

5. To add to what has been said, born and raised in the countryside, depth of the mountain, the habit of eating Japanese food centered on wild vegetables, and the growth history of having graduated from elementary school and not being well-educated (she did not like printing after that) may have increased developing dementia.

[Treatment and progress]

1. We tried to keep the environment of the hospital room quiet, avoiding stimulating behavior, and carried out rehabilitation and hospitalization in a friendly manner.

2. Treatment for core symptoms:

Cognitive stimulation therapy (using puzzles, playing cards, etc.), music therapy (applied to cognitive function), and reminiscence method (I tried to raise the patient's self-esteem by asking her to talk about her personal history from childhood to the present) were done.

3. BPSD (dusk syndrome, nocturnal delirium, frequent urination, etc. are relieved, and good night sleep is induced) are considerably ameliorated by improving the environment. Quetiapine was administered concomitantly for BPSD.

4. Main prescription were memantine 20mg 1 tablet after dinner, donepezil 5mg 2 tablets after breakfast, quetiapine 25mg 2 tablets in 2 divided doses (after lunch, after dinner).

She finally transferred to a nursing home on X+145 days. If I summarize including the conclusion, I think you can see that the basis leading to the diagnosis of AD and what led to the diagnosis of AD rather than other dementias is very important. The guidelines are less important for AD. AD guidelines alone are not sufficient to make a diagnosis of AD rather than other dementias. It is important to comprehensively consider the detailed medical history, signs, and symptoms of AD as mentioned at the AD section.

Dementia with Lewy bodies (DLB)

§21 Characteristics and overview of DLB

This is a disease proposed at an international workshop in 1995 based on research by Kosaka K, et al. since 1976 (Department of Psychiatry, Yokohama City University) (Kosaka K, et al: Acta Neuropathol 36: 221, 1976) (Lewy was the first Jewish German to discover Lewy bodies). It has many names: diffuse Lewy body disease (DLBD), dementia with Lewy bodies (DLB), Parkinson disease with dementia (PDD). Parkinson disease (PD) belongs to the same disease spectrum as DLB in most cases. Although different names (such as DLB or PDD) are used depending on the order in which PD and dementia appear, the true form body is the same.

The number of patients is 1/3 of AD. Prognosis is worse than AD. Most of them are considered to be sporadic and hereditary is low, but it cannot be said that they are completely absent (there is no established theory).

This is dementia disease, but lesions spread not only to the brain but also to the spinal cord, esophagus, heart, etc. Lewy bodies, the main component of α-synuclein aggregates, cause lesion in the central nervous system (causes dementia), nigrostriatal lesions (causes Parkinson's symptoms in 30 to 60%), and autonomic nerves, and in autonomic in the system (autonomic symptoms appear), followed by neuronal damage in the various part of the nervous system.

The symptoms are quite characteristic compared to AD. The Ach system is more affected than AD, and the dopamine system is also affected, resulting in PD. DLB dementia and Parkinson's symptoms appeared almost simultaneously. When AD pathology is complicated (common type), dementia is conspicuous and develops around the age of 70. Pure type, which AD pathology is not complicated, develops PD from an early age in the 30s and progresses quickly.

Pathology

Alpha-synuclein is abundantly found in the presynaptic terminals of nerve fibers in normal individuals (it may be related to the maintenance of synaptic function). In this disease, however, it aggregates pathologically to form Lewy bodies, in neuronal cell bodies. Lewy neurites appear in neurites, which appear not only in central nervous system but also in peripheral nerves, resulting in neuronal loss. Lewy neurite appears in cerebral cortex, amygdala, basal nucleus of Meynert, substantia nigra, locus ceruleus, raphe nucleus, dorsal vagal nucleus, medial lateral nucleus and sympathetic ganglion of spinal cord, and hippocampal CA2-3. The spread of lesions is quite different from AD, involving the brainstem, occipital lobe, esophagus, and heart. In the parahippocampal gyrus, a spongy state is caused. Lewy spheroids appear in the central nucleus of the amygdala and molecular layer of the hippocampus.

Macroscopically, the cerebral cortex and hippocampus show mild atrophy, and in the brainstem, depigmentation of the substantia nigra and the locus ceruleus can be seen. In addition, the Lewy body is seen in the lower part of the esophagus,

It appears in the nerve plexus of the esophageal sphincter muscle (muscles do not relax and become achalasia of the esophagus), and also in the heart (related to cardiac sympathetic nerve damage and orthostatic hypotension).

Ach disorders are stronger in DLB than in AD. Impairment of the substantia nigra causes impairment of the dopamine system, and impairment of the locus ceruleus and raphe nucleus also impairs the noradrenaline and serotonin systems. Alpha-synuclein lesions are associated with 50% of AD, that is, DLB is very closely related to PD and AD.

Why does α-synuclein cause cytotoxicity?

Alpha-synuclein is highly concentrated in axon terminals and is involved in the control of neurotransmitter release (it is said). A related gene, SNCA (4q-21), causes PD. When this α-synuclein polymerizes for some reason to form an oligomer (which is harmful), synaptic dysfunction occurs as follows.

This oligomer is degraded by the chaperone-mediated autophagy (CMA) mechanism of lysosomes, but if it cannot be degraded by CMA due to overproduction of α-synuclein or abnormalities in the SNCA gene and accumulates in the cell, it will load the lysosomes. It also inhibits the degradation of unnecessary proteins. Chaperones in intracellular lysosomes and endoplasmic reticulum bind to unfolded (denatured) proteins and help them to fold properly (native state). After folding is completed, it is released from the bond with the substrate and does not become a part of the substrate after folding. Also, the structure of the chaperone does not change before and after the reaction.

Excess α-synuclein in nerve terminals is released into the synaptic cleft by exocytosis and taken up into postsynapses, causing successive neuronal injury. In addition to such lysosomal stress, mitochondrial stress is also thought to occur, causing cell injury and apoptosis.

§22 Cognitive dysfunction in DLB

What does cognitive dysfunction in DLB look like? It shows progressive cortical and subcortical cognitive dysfunction (described later). Cognitive function decline begins with memory impairment, but the degree of memory impairment is milder than AD. Memory regeneration disorder is the main memory impairment of DLB and is caused by frontal lobe origin, not medial temporal lobe. It is difficult to distinguish from AD when it progresses. In DLB, executive function and problem-solving abilities are more deteriorated than in AD, and symptoms derived from frontal and parietal lobe dysfunction such as attention deficit, configuration disorder, and visuospatial disorder are conspicuous. For this reason, simple tests such as MMSE shows a relatively high score in the early stages, but often presents with various social or occupational difficulties within society. With AD, there is delayed recall disorder while attention and concentration are relatively preserved. With DLB, all indices are low. AD indicates cortical dementia, while DLB indicates a mixture of cortical and subcortical dementia.

Unlike other dementias, one of the characteristics of DLB is fluctuation in cognitive impairment. Cognitive function fluctuates, that is, fluctuations in attention, clarity, and alertness levels, excessive daytime sleepiness, and transient confusion upon awakening. It is often conspicuous in the early stages, occurs relatively rapidly, and may show diurnal fluctuations of minutes to hours, or fluctuations over weeks to months.

Recurrent visual hallucinations are also a core feature of DLB. Typical hallucinations often involve people, small animals, or insects. For example, there are many small children who sit on the side of the bed and stare at the patient. He has complaints about small animals such as insects and snakes crawling on walls and floors. In addition to living creatures, there are many complaints of visual hallucinations such as water, light rays, strings and lint. Visual hallucinations in DLB tend to occur in conjunction with fluctuation in cognition when attention and arousal levels are low, or during dim hours such as in the evening. In some cases, the patient may be aware that it is a hallucination when confirmed during the medical examination. Differentiation from delirium-induced hallucinations is distinguished by the fact that the hallucinations in DLB are persistent and recurrent, and that the patient is able to explain the details of the hallucinations later to family members and doctors. Visual cognitive impairments include optical illusions such as pareidolia (recognizing clothes hanging on a hanger as a person), metamorphopsia (the shape and size of an object changes while looking at it), simulacra phenomenon (recognizing a human face when there are three dots), etc.

Other psychiatric symptoms of DLB are as follows.

Delusional misperceptions are often accompanied with visual hallucinations. "The person on TV is real. The event on TV is happening in my room," "Someone (already dead, stranger, thief, etc.) is there." There are many misidentification delusions related to visual cognition disorder. For instance, the patient claim "I am not at home" though he is at home. "I mistake my wife's face for someone else," "My wife and the impostor have been replaced." are visual cognition disorder. Auditory hallucination is infrequent. Visual hallucination is usually not accompanied by voices or sounds. Pentagon copying is worse than AD patients. Forty % of DLB have major depressive episodes. The incidence of depression in DLB is significantly higher than in AD.

DLB is often seen with PD symptoms. DLB is characterized by the presence of PD symptoms in many cases. Parkinsonism may also be observed in other dementias. Twenty five~fifty % of DLB patients have parkinsonism, which is the most common. There is no big difference from general PD, but symmetric muscle rigidity and bradykinesia are the main feature (tremor is often not noticeable), and tremor at action and myoclonus are sometimes observed. As it progresses, postural reflex disorder and gait disturbance appear, and together with attention disturbance, the risk of falling accidents increases. In addition, vertical eye movement disorder may be observed (must be differentiated from progressive supranuclear palsy).

REM sleep behavior disorder is characteristic of DLB. Under the circumstance of REM sleep, the brain is active and the body is resting. Skeletal muscles are relaxed, and eye movements are active, autonomic nerves are unstable and dreaming. Normally, the dorsolateral nucleus of the pons, the lateral dorsal tegmental nucleus, and the anterior locus ceruleus nucleus inhibit and relax skeletal muscle. In DLB, the muscle tone is not suppressed during RBD and does not relax, so abnormal behaviors that correspond to the content of the dream (such as shouting, hitting the sleeping spouse, etc.) may occur. RBD often precede visual hallucinations and PD. It is a common symptom in the same synucleinopathies as DLB (PD and multiple system atrophy).

Hypersensitivity to antipsychotics is a very characteristic symptoms. Hypersensitivity to antipsychotics is characteristic of DLB and is present in one-third to one-half of cases of DLB. It may cause worsening of PD, disturbance of consciousness, and malignant syndrome even with a small amount of use.

Autonomic nerve injury is also characteristic. Autonomic symptoms such as constipation, neurogenic bladder, and orthostatic hypotension are similar to PD but more frequent than PD. Some patients present with autonomic failure from the beginning. Autonomic failure is dangerous because it can cause falls and fainting.

What are the characteristic radiological findings of DLB? Ventricular enlargement on MRI and the degree of white matter hyperintensity on T2-weighted images are similar to AD. In comparison with AD, medial temporal atrophy is milder than AD. SPECT shows hypoperfusion in the occipital lobe, but the blood flow of the posterior cingulate gyrus is maintained (referred to as the cingulate island sign). PET also demonstrates reduced glucose metabolism in the occipital lobe. 123I-MIBG myocardial scintigraphy which investigates MIBG uptake shows no myocardial uptake due to autonomic nerve distribution disorder. Dopamine transporter (DAT) imaging examines the distribution of dopamine transporters in the striatum demonstrating the degeneration and loss of dopamine neurons.

Summary of clinical course of DLB

1. The first symptoms, in descending order of frequency, were cognitive impairment (61%), PD (36%), psychiatric symptoms (18%), and visual hallucinations (13%).
2. Motor symptoms and autonomic neuropathy in DLB progress faster than in PD. The progression of cognitive impairment in DLB is faster than in AD and VD.
3. The average survival time after onset is less than 10 years (shorter than AD), but there are cases of rapid deterioration of symptoms and death within 1-2 years after onset. Aggravating prognostic factors are advanced age, dementia, psychiatric symptoms, and motor symptoms.
4. DLB patients with hypersensitivity to antipsychotics have a mortality rate two to three times higher than those without.

§23 Diagnostic criteria for DLB

Associated problems for diagnosis of DLB;

1. Older onset DLB lacks characteristic symptoms such as visual hallucinations and PD (easily misdiagnosed as AD).
2. Regarding the clinical course of progression of each symptom, DLB is defined as the onset of dementia before the onset of PD or within 1 year after the onset of PD, and PDD is defined as the case where PD precedes dementia for more than 1 year. If there was elapsed time more than a year and diagnosed as PD. It was called the "rule of one year," but there is no essential difference between the two. The distinction between the two is no longer considered important.
3. AD-type pathological findings (amyloid deposits) are often mixed in the brain of DLB (sometimes complicating the diagnosis of DLB). In DLB, both Lewy-related pathology and AD-type pathology contribute to the development of dementia symptoms.

To summarize the clinical diagnostic criteria for DLB (2017): two 1s(①~④), or one 1(①~④) and one 2 (①~③).

1. Core features, the first three typically appear early and persist throughout the clinical course.

① Cognitive fluctuations with marked changes in attention or clarity

② Recurring constructed concrete hallucinations

③ REM sleep behavior disorder that may precede cognitive decline

④ One or more of the following idiopathic parkinsonisms (bradykinesia, bradykinesia, resting tremor, rigidity)

2. Indicative biomarkers

① Decreased uptake of dopamine transporters in the basal ganglia as shown by SPECT or PET

② Decreased uptake in MIBG myocardial scintigraphy

③ Confirmation of REM sleep without hypotonia by polysomnography (McKeith IG, et al : Neurology 89: 1, 2017)

This diagnostic criterion for DLB is considered much more useful than those for AD.

§24 Basic concept of DLB treatment

Currently, there is no fundamental treatment for DLB brain lesions caused by α-synuclein. Treatment for symptoms can be broadly divided into drug therapy and non-drug therapy. Nonpharmacologic therapy consists of care and accommodation, that is, environment arrangement and is more important, but there are few significant studies.

Specific nervous system (dopamine system, Ach system, serotonin system) is disturbed and its symptoms are caused, and drugs are used for it. Symptoms targeted for treatment include cognitive impairment, BPSD such as hallucinations, depression, apathy, sleep disturbances, EPS, and autonomic symptoms. It is necessary to pay close attention to the possibility that treatments which improve one symptom may exacerbate other symptoms, and side effects such as drug hypersensitivity.

Pharmacological treatment

Pharmacological treatment for psychiatric, behavioral symptoms and sleep disorders for DLB are somewhat different from that of AD. In Japan, donepezil is the only cholinesterase inhibitor effective for cognitive impairment in DLB and covered by insurance. Donepezil also helps BPSD such as psycho-motor abnormality, especially hallucination, delusion, excitement, and apathy (Mori E, et al : Ann Neurol 72 :41, 2012). If ineffective, atypical antipsychotics such as quetiapine, olanzapine, risperidone and Yokukansan may be somewhat effective. Galantamine is effective against visual hallucinations. It is known cholinergic side effects such as nausea, vomiting, and anorexia are common, but parkinsonism is described as largely unchanged in most cases and conversely exacerbated (particularly tremor) in some cases of PDD. Clonazepam is effective for RBD. In addition, efficacy of melatonin, Yokukansan, ramelteon, donepezil, etc. has been reported as effective. Quetiapine is covered by health insurance for hallucinations, delusions, and delirium associated with PD. In 2005, the US Food and Drug Administration (FDA) announced that atypical antipsychotics increase the risk of death in elderly people with dementia, and consideration must be given to their use. Typical antipsychotics, however, have equal or much greater risks.

Typical antipsychotic drugs (haloperidol, chlorpromazine, etc.) should be avoided as it shows a high degree of hypersensitivity in DLB. It should be noted that similar reactions may also occur with atypical antipsychotics, which are less likely to cause EPS. The use of SSRIs (selective serotonin reuptake inhibitors) and SNRIs (serotonin noradrenaline reuptake inhibitors) is recommended for depressive symptoms often seen in DLB, but there are no significant studies on their usefulness in DLB. Drugs with anticholinergic effects such as tricyclic antidepressants (Anafranil, Tryptanol, trihexyphenidyl , etc.) should be avoided due to the risk of exacerbation of dementia except for special uses. The use of levodopa is recommended for PD seen in DLB. There is no clear cognitive decline as a side effect, but anti-PD drugs may exacerbate cognitive symptoms, so give care to exacerbation of cognitive symptom and start from small doses. It is less effective than for usual PD. For autonomic symptoms (orthostatic hypotension, constipation): Constipation is managed in the usual way. For orthostatic hypotension, I recommend wearing elastic stockings, taking salt and water, and drug therapy such as midodrine, Florinef, and droxidopa. They are commonly used but there are no significant reports.

§25 Illustrative case of DLB

The patient is 74 year-old female presenting with visual hallucinations and REM sleep behavior disorder.

[Past history] hypertension and angina pectoris at 60 years old,

[Family history] Her husband died 10 years ago and she lives alone. She has two sons. The eldest son's wife is a care manager.

[History of current illness] Recent memory impairment has been noticeable since X-3 years, and it has been progressive, so she sometimes has to stay out at her eldest son's house, and her family has noticed her hallucinations and behavioral abnormalities at night. Thirty days before admission to our hospital, right hemiparesis suddenly appeared. She transferred to a neurosurgery department and underwent endoscopic hematoma evacuation for left frontal subcortical hemorrhage (hematoma weighing 25 g). Her right hemiplegia improved in one week, but she transferred to our hospital on X day at the request of her family, who said "I'm worried about leaving her alone." CT at onset: Subcortical hemorrhage in the left frontal lobe was shown (Fig.9, 1-2). Neither particular lesions other than bleeding nor obvious atrophy (no medial temporal lobe atrophy) was noted.

[Current condition]

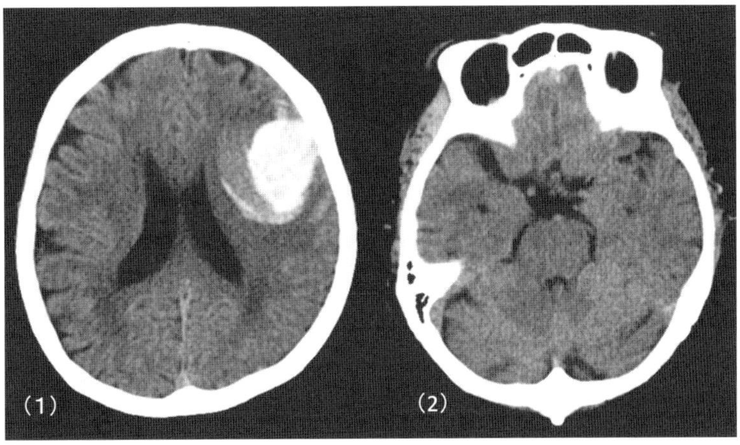

Fig.9. CT at onset: Subcortical hemorrhage was shown in the left frontal lobe (1). She has no particular atrophy from temporal lobe to hippocampal area (2).

<General physical findings> Constipation was persistent and laxatives such as Magnesium oxide (2.0) were administered, but it was insufficient and required glycerin enemas once every 4 days.

<Neurologic findings> She was ambidextrous and showed no aphasia, no Parkinsonism and could walk independently. She showed disorientation (date, place), topographical disorder (cannot go back to her room from the dining room), anosognosia, etc. Her problem-solving ability and executive function are disturbed.

Cognitive function fluctuations: Sudden fluctuations (lasting about 3 hours) in recognition, orientation, and communication, etc., occur once every two weeks.

Symptoms of autonomic nervous system failure: In addition to the aforementioned constipation, fainting attacks thought to be caused by orthostatic hypotension (described later) occur twice a month.

Nocturnal delirium: After dinner, she left the ward at night twice a month at the beginning. She turns on the lights in the middle of the night and open and close the drawers of the shelves in the room many times to start changing clothes (sometimes wearing the jacket inside out).

REM sleep behavior disorder: She gets out of bed at night, opens the curtains around the bed of other patients, and makes loud and incomprehensible talk about the content, and when the staff guides her to her own bed, she will return to her senses and then sleep quietly until morning. This happens once or twice a month.

Visual hallucinations: 2-3 times/week at night before bedtime. "There is a child there, a girl with pigtails, about the second grade of elementary school." She made remarks such as "When I opened the bathroom door, there was a girl."

[Main laboratory findings]

Orthostatic test: Blood pressure decreased from 130/70 to 90/50 by standing up.

Cognitive function tests: MMSE 18 (particularly poor pentagon reproduction), HDS-R 19, Raven color matrix test 14/36 indicates dementia.

BIT behavioral neglect test: In the normal test, 86/146 of line segments, letters, asterisks, copying, and drawing were all below the cutoff, and right hemispatial neglect, visuospatial cognitive impairment, and attention disturbance were observed.

If the severity rating of AD is applied, it was FAST 4, and the degree of BPSD was Behave-AD 34.

[Diagnosis/differential diagnosis]

According to the Clinical diagnostic criteria for DLB (McKeith IG, 2017), her condition met three core features for probable DLB: visual hallucinations, fluctuating cognitive function, and REM sleep behavior abnormalities. This case was complicated by subcortical hemorrhage during the course of DLB, but did not show clear symptoms of cerebrovascular dementia.

[Treatment policy/plan]

She had a care manager in his family who understands this disease well. As a result of discussing her future policies, she gave up living alone in the future. As a non-pharmacological treatment, her family expected that auditory hallucinations, visual hallucinations, and insomnia at night could be improved by improving the environment of the ward. She tried to stay out overnight for her strong will but her family experienced exhaustion due to problems such as locking doors, fires, operating water faucets, difficulty paying attention to signals and railroad crossings outdoors, and behavioral abnormalities at night. After that, we made an environment improvement that encourages dialogue with the roommates.

[Treatment/ prescription]

Consent was not obtained for the use of antidementia drugs. Nocturnal delirium and visual hallucinations are symptoms that burden the patient, and consent was obtained for the use of atypical antipsychotics. There was no overreaction to antipsychotics, and these symptoms were relieved. Clonazepam 1 mg, which is said to be the first choice for REM sleep behavior disorder, was started and maintained at 2 mg. Symptoms disappeared and clonazepam was discontinued 3 months later. The improvement of BPSD was thought to be largely related to the successful communication with patients in the same room and the successful preparation of the environment.

[Progress/response to problems]

Both the core symptoms and BPSD were significantly improved. Then, it was considered possible to live with the eldest son's family (a family of four) at home after discharge. She was discharged from the hospital on 6 months after the onset to his eldest son's house.

To summarize briefly, I hope you have understood that the characteristics are very different from AD, and the diagnostic criteria are very meaningful, unlike AD.

Vascular dementia

§26 General characteristics of vascular dementia

Vascular dementia (VD) is caused by cerebrovascular disease that appears within 3 months after the onset of cerebrovascular disease, and is the second most common dementia after AD.

Naturally, it has the distinct feature that the imaging findings are consistent with the neurological findings. VD merges AD at 25.7% (Jellinger KA, et al: Acta Neuropathol 119: 421, 2010). When VD is combined with AD, the incidence of dementia becomes more than doubles, and the life prognosis is said to be poor. Four antidementia drugs are recommended, but may be mediated by effects on comorbid AD. Basically, they are not effective on VD itself.

The characteristic symptoms in order of incidence are:

1. Gait disorder (PD-like brachybasia, tendency to fall).
2. Dysuria (frequent urination, urgency, urinary incontinence).
3. Pseudobulbar palsy (dysphagia, dysarthria).
4. Severe depression (feeling very depressed).
5. Subcortical dementia (described later).
6. Emotional incontinence, affective disorder (emotional instability, anxiety, sleep disturbance, delirium, apathy, excitement).
7. Spotted dementia (symptoms change depending on the day and time of day and are unstable. Feeling fine in the morning, but depressed in the afternoon, etc.).
8. Executive dysfunction or attention deficit (difficulty maintaining attention at work, increasing mistakes and slow reaction, poor organization, low spontaneity, low motivation). These are symptoms that are frequently encountered on a daily basis when examining patients in the ward.

There are various diagnostic criteria, but NINDS-AIREN is the strictest diagnostic criteria (Roman GC, et al: Neurology 43: 250, 1993). However, what is universally stated in any criterion are:

1. Lesions clearly caused by cerebrovascular disease.
2. Dementia onset within 3 months of onset.
3. Presence of dementia: In addition to memory impairment, execution disorder, language disorder, visuospatial cognitive disorder, complex attention disorder (persistence, distributiveness, selectivity, processing speed), social cognitive disorder (coarse social behavior). Two or more impairments as mentioned above are found.

Classification comprising multiple infarction with dementia (atherothrombotic, cardiogenic cerebral embolism), small vessel disease (lacuna infarction) with dementia, hypoperfusion, strategic single infarct dementia, hemorrhage with dementia, etc. are shown in NINDS-AIREN diagnostic criteria (Roman GC, et al: Neurology 43: 250, 1993). From the perspective of staff who often encounter stroke clinically, it is a natural classification. Although I will omit describing general clinical facts, I will only mention Binswanger disease and CADASIL for reference.

Binswanger disease

It causes extensive and diffuse demyelination of the cerebral white matter and presents with progressive and severe dementia. In every case, circulatory disturbance in the perforator region causes widespread ischemia and damage to white matter fibers, resulting in fragmentation of prefrontal cortex circuits (prefrontal cortex, caudate nucleus, globus pallidum, thalamus) and thalamocortical tracts (knee of internal capsule, anterior limb of internal capsule, anterior part of centrum semiovale, and corona radiate). Subcortical dementia appears due to severe disruption of white matter in those areas. Microscopically, there is diffuse and severe demyelination of the white matter, conspicuous in the periventricular area, corona radiata, and centrum semiovale, but the axons are relatively preserved (Fig.10). In most cases, the progression is slow, with executive dysfunction, slow thinking, depression, and emotional incontinence, but capacity of memory is relatively well maintained. Neurological symptoms include motor paralysis, pseudobulbar palsy (morbid tearful smile, dysarthria, dysphagia), cerebrovascular parkinsonism (frozen gait, brachybasia, akinesia, muscle rigidity), tendon hyperreflexia, pathological reflexes, coordination disorder, overactive bladder (frequent urination, urinary incontinence), etc.

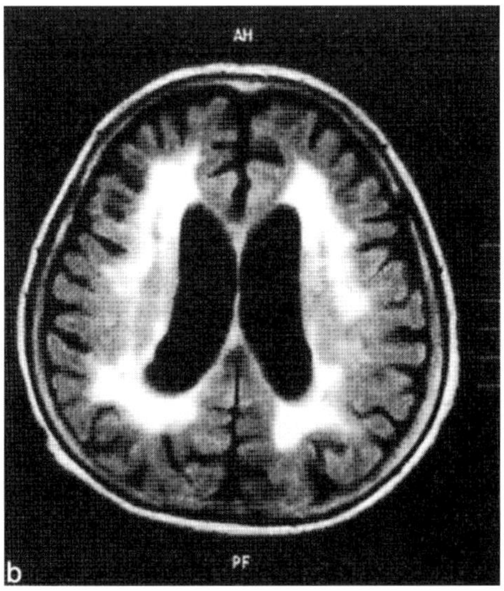

Fig.10. FLAIR MRI shows high intensity area extending wide area of the bilateral subcortex, indicating ischemic degeneration of Binswanger disease.

CADASIL , CARASIL

CADASIL is abbreviation of cerebral autosomal dominant arteriopathy with subcortical infarcts and leukoencephalopathy. It is juvenile (40-60 years old) cerebral vascular disease caused by autosomal dominant inheritance (nucleotide sequence mutation of NOTCH 3 gene). The patient has headache from the young age. Degenerative findings are caused by impaired circulation of periventricular white matter. The characteristic is cerebral infarction around the temporal horn of the lateral ventricle. Microscopically, accumulation of granular osmiophilic material in arteriolar media is observed resulting in disturbance of vascular reactivity (it is called vessel ducting).

CARASIL is abbreviation of cerebral autosomal recessive arteriopathy with subcortical infarcts and leukoencephalopathy. It is caused by autosomal recessive inheritance (HTRA1 gene mutation). The patient shows baldness by age 30, gait disturbance from 20s, spondylolisthesis, and low back pain.

What is subcortical dementia in general?

It is observed in PSP, VD, Binswanger's disease, PD, CBD, etc. Symptoms caused by disorders in the dorsolateral prefrontal cortex is similar to the symptoms caused by the subcortical lesion occupying wide area except for the frontal lobe, (but mainly including frontal lobe). The symptoms show executive dysfunction, motor program abnormalities, decreased motivation, decreased spontaneity, emotional flattening, lethargy, bradyphrenia, depression, and apathy. Normally, white matter lesions are not responsible for neurological symptoms bur symptoms appear when the spread or intensity of damage exceeds a certain threshold. In more detail:

1. Impaired ability to manipulate and effectively utilize existing knowledge according to the situation, impaired integration of cognitive functions, impaired recall of learned knowledge.
2. Decrease in thought process and information processing speed.
3. Not the loss of memory, but a type of escaping of his memory that cannot recall immediately.
4. Personality and emotional disorders such as acathexis,

apathy, apathy, childishness, lack of control, and anger attacks.
5. Impaired attention, impaired motivation.

What is the difference from cerebral cortical dementia (typically AD)? Subcortical dementia is a type of dementia in which cognitive functions are relatively preserved but there is a problem in the ability to activate them, and resembles frontal lobe symptoms.

§27 Let's give a representative case of VD.

The patient is 85-year-old female presenting with left hemiplegia, memory impairment and dementia.
[Past history] Atrial fibrillation.
[Family history] Her husband died 17 years ago.
[Present illness] Since two years before admission, she had marked forgetfulness.

Twenty days before admission to our hospital, left hemiparesis appeared and she was admitted to a neurosurgery department. Diffusion images of her MRI showed high density in her right frontotemporal lobe, confirming occlusion of her right internal carotid artery on MRA (Fig.11). She underwent endovascular surgery with a diagnosis of cardiogenic cerebral embolism, which allowed recanalization 2 hours and 50 minutes after her onset. Her left hemiplegia improved slightly. She transferred to our hospital for rehabilitation on X day.
[Current condition]

<Neurologic findings> Left hemiplegia (MMT: 4/5 for both upper and lower limbs), left body neglect, apraxia (she needed assistance to change clothes because she tries to put on the left and right reversely), urinary incontinence, and frequent urination were seen. In addition, the following cognitive symptoms were present. As core symptoms, disorientation (time and place) and recent memory impairment were prominent.

BPSD are as follows:

After 5 p.m., her depression worsened along with anxiety, and she became paranoid and agitated (depressive symptoms, dusk syndrome). Statements such as "I was scared when the nurse threw me a towel. Why is she malicious?" She had strong paranoia such as "I was treated unethically. Evil will perish. I am sad to be betrayed by a nurse (persecutory delusions)."

Agitation from before dinner until midnight is striking.

Refusal of nursing care and violent behavior such as hitting the caregiver when helping with dressing or toileting. Desire to go home appeared often in the evening. Delusions about being stolen such as "My bag was stolen" were sometimes observed, then we looked for it together, and she could understand the situation.
[Neurological examination]: MMSE 17/30, HDS-R 15/30 (impaired orientation to time, date, season, etc., immediate recall, delayed recall, arithmetic disturbance, drawing of the cube, etc., indicating generalized cognitive decline).

Trail making test: TMT-A marked attentional decline taking 300 seconds. TMT-B took too long and was discontinued because it was impossible to continue the test (executive dysfunction). Miyake memorization test

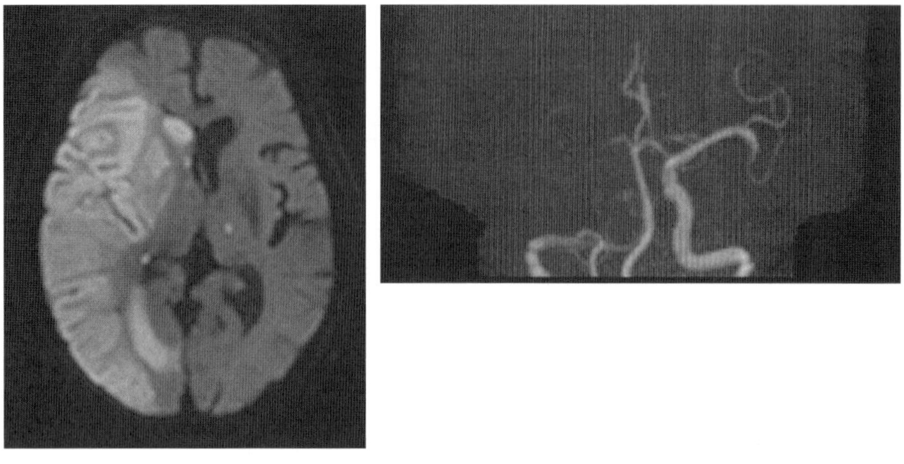

Fig.11. Diffusion MRI (1) and MRA (2) show right temporo-parietal lobe infarction caused by right internal carotid artery occlusion.

showed severe attention deficit. Frontal assessment battery: Executive dysfunction (7/18).

BIT behavioral neglect test: 87/146 on normal test. Left hemispatial neglect (letters, asterisks, line segment deletion, etc.) was observed. Not only ignorance, but also attention disorders were basically seen.

[Diagnosis and differential diagnosis] Dementia is obvious in the DSM-5 dementia diagnostic criteria (2013). In the AHA/ASA diagnostic criteria for vascular cognitive impairment (Gorelick PB, et al: Stroke 42 : 2672, 2011), among three areas of dementia such as performance impairment/attention impairment, memory, and visuospatial cognitive function, impairment of activities of daily living was observed in the cognitive domain. A definitive diagnosis was obtained because there was a clear temporal linkage between the presence of cerebrovascular disease findings and the onset of cognitive impairment.

[Treatment/main prescription] Warfarin 1 mg 2 tablets after breakfast. Quetiapine 25mg 3 tablets (1 tablet after lunch, 2 tablets after dinner).

[Treatment and progress/response to problems] She is able to walk 10m freehand (proximal monitoring). By using quetiapine, anxiety, persecution delusions, delirium, frequent urination, etc. have improved to the extent that they do not interfere with her life in the ward. Antidementia drugs could not be administered because the family could not agree to the possibility of the appearance of circulatory and digestive side effects. Three months after admission she transferred to a nursing home.

In summary, I have presented my experienced case of typical VD. Clinical course such as onset within 3 months after apoplexy, characteristic symptoms such as frequent urination, severe depressive state, subcortical dementia, emotional disturbance, not only memory but also executive function, attention deficit, visuospatial cognitive impairment could lead to a definitive diagnosis. You can see that this is a typical characteristic case.

Fronto-temporal lobar degeneration (FTLD)

§28 Characteristics and overview of FTLD

FTLD is a group of characteristic diseases with lesions in the frontotemporal lobe and sometimes in the parietal lobe. Compared to other dementias, the symptoms of FTLD are very strange and exhibit distinctive positive symptoms that stand out. Behavioral abnormalities, aphasia, and dementia are main symptoms. Tau, TDP, FUS, etc. appear primarily in neurons, and lesions of characteristic ranges appears in the frontotemporal and sometimes in the parietal lobes. The number of patients with FTLD is currently 12,000 in Japan, and almost all of them are sporadic, while hereditary accounts for 30-50% in Europe and the United States. Abnormalities in the C9orf72 gene are the most common in FTLD. Other details on frequency are unknown. FTLD accounts for less than 5% of dementia.

There is no effective treatment and the prognosis is poor in most cases. Many patients who have not been diagnosed with FTLD are referred from departments other than neurology or psychiatry, that is, you have to be careful about patients referred directly from orthopedic, emergency medicine, internal medicine, and surgical departments.

Understanding the neuropathological classification makes it difficult to grasp for non-FTLD basic researchers. Therefore, that is not very familiar. It was classified basically by McKhann et al. in 2001, based on the presence or absence of inclusion bodies and their components such as tau protein (Spillantini MG, et al: Proc Natl Acad Sci USA 95: 7737, 1998), TAR DNA-binding protein of 43KD (TDP-43), ubiquitin, and fused in sarcoma (FUS) (Table 2). Tau protein is one of the microtubule-associated proteins, and is further classified into 3-repeat tau and 4-repeat tau according to the repeat number of the microtubule-associated region on the C-terminal side (McKhann GM, et al: Arch Neurol 58:1803, 2001). Due to space limitations, I will not discuss the academic transition that led to the current neuropathological classification. Please refer to the following for details (Dementia Textbook: Japanese Dementia Society 2014) (Clinical study of frontotemporal dementia: Ikeda M, Nakayama Shoten, Japan 2010).

§29 Clinical classification of FTLD

Clinical classification in FTLD was done according to the affected areas of brain in FTLD (atrophy, decline of cerebral blood flow and metabolism). FTLDs generally

Table 2.Neuropathological classification of FTLD

MAPT: microtubule-associated protein tau, PGRN : progranulin, VCP: valosin-containing protein, CHAMP 2B: charged multivesicular body protein 2B, FTLD-U: frontotemporal lobar degeneration with ubiquitinated inclusions, DLDH: dementia lacking distinctive histology (Cairns NJ: Acta Neuropathol 114: 5, 2007) (McKhann GM: Arch Neurol 58: 1803, 2001)

	Classification by Cairns 2007		Classification by McKhann 2001
	constituent protein, inclusion body	disease	disease
FTLD-tau (tauopathy)	group 1 3 repeat tau dominant	FTLD with Pick body FTLD with MAPT mutation	Pick disease FTLD-17
	group 2 4 repeat tau dominant	Corticobasal degeneration Progressive supranuclear palsy Argyrophilic grain disease Sporadic multiple system tauopathy with dementia FTLD with MAPT mutation	CBD PS FTLD-17
	group 3 3,4 repeat tau	FTLD with MAPT mutation NFTD	FTLD-17 NFTD
FTLD without inclusions	group 4 tau and ubiquitin negative	Dementia lacking distinctive histology Progressive subcortical gliosis	DLDH
TDP-43 proteinopathy (FTLD-U)	group 5 tau negative, ubiquitin positive (TDP-43 positive)	FTLD-U with MND(FTLD-U type 1～3) FTLD-U without MND(FTLD-U type 1～3) FTLD-U with PGRN mutation(FTLD-U type 3) FTLD-U with VCP mutation(FTLD-U type4) FTLD-U associated with 9th gene(FTLD-U type 2)	FTLD-U with MND FTLD-U without MND
FTLD with other type inclusions	group 6 ubiquitin positive TDP-43 negative tau negative	FTLD-U with CHAMP2B mutation Basophilic inclusion body disease(BIBD)	FTLD-FUS
	group 7 ubiquitin,α-internexin positive inclusion body	neuronal intermediate filament inclusion disease (NIFID)	

deteriorate cerebral blood flow (CBF) and metabolism followed by atrophy. Clinical classification differs from the neuropathological classification. Affected areas of brain in FTLD are shown in Fig.12.

1. Progressive non-fluent aphasia (PNFA)

Atrophy of the left central gyrus, left inferior~middle frontal lobe, and island are seen. PNFA is characterized by grammatical errors (53% of PNFA has agrammar) and speech apraxia (94% of PNFA shows speech apraxia). Histologically it accounts for tau in 50% and AD in 31%.

2. Behavioral variant of frontotemporal dementia (bvFTD)

Atrophy and decreased CBF was observed in the frontal lobe and anterior part of temporal lobe, more specifically the rostral limbic system of the anterior and medial temporal lobe, frontal lobe and anterior part of temporal lobe, the anterior cingulate gyrus, ventromedial frontal cortex, ventral striatum, amygdala, anterior part of insular cortex, and rostral limbic system such as anterior and medial temporal regions. There is no left-right difference.

BvFTD is classified into 3 types: (1) apallic type (apathy, indifference, decreased spontaneity), (2) stereotypic type (stereotypic behavior, compulsive behavior, perseverance), and (3) disinhibition type showing anti-social behavior and leaving behavior, the main symptom of which is behavioral abnormalities rather than language. Stereotypic behavior can be seen 95% of bvFTD. Histologically, tau accounted for 42% and TDP accounted for 30%.

3. Semantic dementia (SD), semantic variant primary progressive aphasia (svPPA)

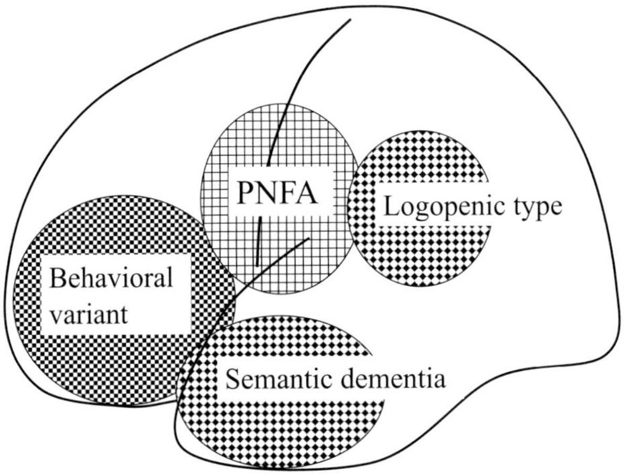

Fig.12. Schematic drawing of left side view indicating affected area with decrease of CBF and metabolism in the FTLD brain.

Asymmetric atrophic lesions in the anterior temporal lobe and the inferior temporal gyrus are seen and are often on the left side, but sometimes on the right side, and eventually become bilateral.

SD is characterized by language impairment rather than behavior impairment, but stereotypic behavior is also very many and can be seen 72% of SD. It presents with symptoms such as difficulty in naming goods, difficulty in pronouncing words, difficulty in remembering (recollecting) words, difficulty in understanding words (the name of the thing the patients are trying to say does not appear), and inability to point to objects among multiple objects (recognition disorder). I showed a patient a pencil ("empitsu" in Japanese) and asked him what he said. He couldn't answer, so I gave a hint that it was an "enpi・・," and he answered "Oh, it is an enpi." Fluency is preserved and repetition is preserved. Grammar is preserved, but in parrot return (echo language). The dumpling (Japanese sweet rice ball called "dango" is read as danshi (we Japanese never says "danshi", but for surface aphasia he says "danshi." Similarly, the partner (Aite in Japanese) is read as "soushi" (surface aphasia). Crescent moon (Mikazuki in Japanese) is spoken as "Sankazuki." Complementary phenomenon (described in the next page) is famous in SD.

Forty-seven % of SD patients have prosopagnosia. In patients with right-sided atrophy, they cannot recognize the faces of celebrities or family members, nor recognize famous buildings such as Kinkakuji Temple (the most famous temple in Kyoto that every Japanese knows) or Tokyo Tower. It doesn't show any sense that he has already known or seen. Even if he sees a famous person, he can't recognize who he is.

Histologically, TDP-43 accounts for 68%, and tau or AD account for 16%.

4. Logopenic variant primary progressive aphasia (LvPPA)

Posterior part of left temporal lobe to parietal lobe is affected. LvPPA is mainly characterized by language impairment rather than behavior, and, as the meaning of logo (words) and penic (few) means, there is little expression of language. It shows word recall disorder (all patients with LvPPA has word recall disorder), repetition disorder, and phonological paraphasia. Histologically, it is identical with AD.

In addition, the characteristics of the detailed localization of the lesion (atrophy site) are as follows.

Tauopathy (group1-3): atrophy of the medial temporal lobe.

DNTC, argyrophilic granulopathy (AGD) in Group 2: severe atrophy of temporal lobe, enlargement of cisterna ambiens.

Group 3, neurofibrillary tangle dementia (NFTD): marked atrophy of posterior part of temporal lobe.

Chromosome 9-linked FTLD-U in group 5: atrophy in the anterior temporal lobe, atrophy of parietal lobe, occipital lobe, and cerebellum.

FTLD-U with PGRN mutations in group 5: bilateral medial temporal lobe atrophy but asymmetric.

§30 Various speech symptoms in FTLD

In FTLD, various symptoms of aphasia appear due to the presence of lesions in the frontotemporal lobe. The symptoms of aphasia are subtly different because each localization of language area is subtly different.

Difficulty in word finding and anonymity; the patients express "Fusuma (in Japanese)" as "Open and enter the sliding door." It may be similar to amnestic aphasia

Poor spontaneous speech, difficulty in repetition, paraphasias, and misreadings.

Amnestic aphasia (anonymous aphasia): Difficulty in word finding, impaired naming, nouns are often impaired. It is recognized in every type of FTLD.

Impaired word recall (inability to name objects) and impaired recognition (inability to point to a designated object from multiple objects).

Repetitive language: Repeating the same word.

Surface aphasia: It is recognized in every type of FTLD except bvFTD (described in the section of SD in the previous page).

Pure word dumbness: Mandarin orange (mikan in Japanese) → "mi ・ ・kan." "mi ・ ・ka ・ ・nn."

Speech apraxia: It is frequently seen in PNFA, also in logopenic type of FTLD. Difficulty in starting words and sentence, choppy, distorted articulation, and speech with prosody disturbances are observed. It is a famous example sentence; "I don't have a positive attitude when talking to customers" is expressed as "I ・ d, d, do not h have a po ・ po sitive an atti ・ ・ tude."

Agrammatical: Omission of functional words such as particles and auxiliary verbs is observed. For instance, "Tomorrow, school, I go." It is frequently recognized in PNFA.

Paragrammatical: There are correct verbs and function words, but the words and grammar are used incorrectly. For example, "I'll go to school"→ "School go to tomorrow."

Persistent language (stay language): No matter what you ask, he repeats relatively same long speeches or same words. He inserts the same words and phrases such as one's name and date of birth during conversation.

Phonological paraphasia: phone (Denwa in Japanese)→ phone (Densu), dog (Inu in Japanese)→dog (Chinu), pencil (Empitsu in Japanese)→pencil (Kanpichi).

Verbal paraphasia: (mispronunciation of words) dog→-cat, car →airplane

Graphical paraphasia: (Spectacles) Megane→Megare.

Illusion: egg (Tamago in Japanese)→egg (Tanago).

Response language: The patients answer my question as it is. He parrots back what the other person said.

Perseveration: The patient repeats what he has said.

Music box clock symptom: The patients always talk about the same topic.

Complementary phenomenon: It is frequently observed in SD. Every Japanese knows Japanese popular proverb "If the dogs walks, it hits the stick." The examiner says "If the dog walks" but even if the patient is asked not to say the next phrase, the patient answers "it hit the stick." He is forced to continue the next phrase reluctantly.

§31 Pick's disease

It is the most famous classic disease of FTLD and was first reported in 1892 by Arnold Pick of Czechoslovakia. The first case was: A 71-year-old man with onset of forgetfulness showed occasional fainting attacks, delirium, domestic violence, language abnormalities, incomprehension of language and letters, inability to name objects, and incomprehensibility of letters and writing. He died of pneumonia one month after hospitalization. There was marked atrophy of the frontotemporal lobe.

Pick reported macroscopic findings of the brain at autopsy, with relative preservation of the superior temporal gyrus and marked atrophy of the frontal lobe and middle-lower temporal gyrus. In 1906, German Alois Alzheimer (advocate Alzheimer's disease) reported histopathologically that Pick-like gynecocytes and Pick-like mast cells were observed. Currently, Pick's disease is defined as a disease characterized by marked atrophy of the frontotemporal lobes, Pick-like gynecocytes, Pick cells (ballooned neurons), and belongs to group 1 with tauopathy. In Japan, there is almost no heritability, and familial occurrence is rare, while 1/3 in Europe and the United States are autosomal dominant (Rosso SM, et al: Brain 126: 2016, 2003). Pick's disease is less common than CBD and PSP.

§32 Elderly onset tauopathy

There is a group of diseases called primary age-related tauopathy (PART). This is a group of diseases in which neurofibrillary tangles become prominent with age and dementia becomes evident.

Neurofibrillary tangle senile dementia (NFTD, SD-NFT)

There is no senile plaque. Neurofibrillary tangle (NFT) causes dementia. In hippocampus and parahippocampal gyrus, massive NFTs, neuropil threads and neuronal loss are observed. Medial temporal lobe atrophy is predominantly posterior. The main symptoms are memory impairment and disorientation, and other cognitive symptoms do not appear unless the patient is very old.

Argyrophilic grain dementia (AGD)

It is often associated and combined with CBD, AD, and DLB. Dementia is caused by argyrophilic granules. Medial temporal lobe atrophy is anteriorly dominant and bilaterally asymmetrical (it spreads from the detour gyrus to the medial temporal lobe to the limbic system, and these become atrophy). Ninety-seven percent of AGD patients show MCI, which is milder than AD. Memory impairment is the main symptom, and other symptoms are relatively rare. The cognition function is relatively maintained (emotional changes such as aggression, personality changes, irritability, delusions, sullenness, agitation, apathy, etc. are sometimes present).

Corticobasal degeneration (CBD)

CBD shows, if anything, cortical dementia not subcortical dementia. This is also known as Pick's disease type 2 and sporadic. Various parts of the cerebrum and the basal ganglia are affected, but the substantia nigra is most affected. Both neurons and glia are affected; For example, astrocytic plaques in the cerebral cortex, swollen neurons, threads in the cortical white matter, and oligodendroglial coiled bodies are seen. Morphological changes are more advanced than PSP. Frontoparietal lobe atrophy has crosswise difference.

Onset is from the upper extremities. Clumsy upper extremities, ideomotor apraxia (impairment of pantomime, that is, he can use comb to comb hair but cannot imitate combing without holding comb, which also seen in AD). Alien hand sign (the patient's hand interferes with the movements of the other hand against his will), structural apraxia, cortical dementia in the advanced stage, supranuclear oculomotor disorder, parkinsonian symptoms, myoclonus, executive function disorders, disinhibition, and other personality changes, and non-fluent aphasia are characteristic.

Limb kinetic apraxia (it is caused by central gyrus injury, showing clumsiness and weakness of contralateral upper extremity, inability to press buttons, difficulty of picking up coins), asymmetry of apraxia, muscle stiffness, etc. are also characteristic. Depression is common but PSP-like affective disturbances, hallucinations, delusions, delirium, confusion-like states are rare.

Tau is composed of paired helical filaments (PHF) and straight filaments, which form the neurofibrillary tangles that appear in AD brains. Tau accumulates also in the brain of many neurodegenerative diseases including Pick's disease, CBD, PSP and AGD. In AD, tau accumulates mainly in neurons, whereas in Pick's disease, PSP, CBD, and AGD, tau accumulates not only in neurons but also in glial cells.

Progressive supranuclear palsy (PSP)

It shows autosomal dominant inheritance. In the cerebral cortex, the frontal lobe is affected. PSP-type NFTs, tuft-shaped astrocytes, glial fibrillary tangles in neurons, and tau protein abnormalities in also glial cells are observed. Highly educated is a risk factor. CBD and PSP are related diseases, and frequency CBD : PSP is 1: 2.6.

Subcortical dementia or frontal lobe dementia (slow thinking, impulsiveness, perseveration, persistence), personality change, apathy, affective disorder, memory disorder, imitative behavior, degraded personality, episodic stupor, hallucination, delusion are observed.

Neurologically, the patients show pyramidal tract signs, axial rigidity (rigidity is stronger in the neck and trunk than in the extremities), nuchal dystonia (nuchal flexion in the terminal stage), tendency to fall (backward), supranuclear oculomotor palsy (downward gaze paralysis), Parkinsonism, paradoxical gait (the patient is improved by overcoming an obstacle in front of a frozen leg forward), applause sign (the patient claps his hands 3 times but can't stop and he keeps going and clap 4 times), and cerebellar ataxia symptoms, etc. LvPPA and SD are primary progressive aphasia, in which dementia is not very noticeable at first, but gradually progresses to dementia. In both PSP and CBD, dementia is not noticeable in the early stages, but dementia progresses as the disease progresses, and they are a famous discases in neurology due to various neurological symptoms. PSP shows subcortical dementia. The humming bird sign is famous for midbrain atrophy on MRI.

Diffuse neurofibrillary tangle disease

Diffuse neurofibrillary tangles with calcification (DNTC) is a disease that is more common in presenile women than elderly women. It shows presenile onset aged 40 to 60 years, male : female ratio 1:3. It shows NFT positive tau staining with severe neuronal loss, and mixture of PHF, straight tubule and neuropil threads with highly widespread distribution in the cerebral cortex. Frontal and temporal lobes are atrophic. Calcification (Ca, P, lead deposits) in the basal ganglia and dentate nucleus is Fahr disease-like. No senile spot is observed.

The patients develop memory impairment and exhibits cortical dementia. The disease is characterized by AD-like memory impairment and the coexistence of Pick'disease like personality changes. They present personality changes as mentioned above, hallucinations, delusions, disinhibition, behavioral abnormalities, spontaneous hypoactivity, parkinsonism, and language disorders such as amnestic aphasia and sensory aphasia, etc.

§33 What are the symptoms of FTLD in general?

Common manifestation mechanisms in FTLD is different from AD. Unlike AD, the posterior part of the brain is preserved, so in the early stages there are no problems with ADL itself. Behavioral and psychotic abnormalities derived from the frontal lobe dysfunction itself appear, because inhibition against limbic system, basal ganglia and the posterior part of the brain is unlinked.

Symptoms that are likely to appear from the early stage include changes in social behavior, emotions, and daily life, decreased spontaneity, depressive state, stereotyped behavior, loss of interest in society, loss of interest in self, disinhibition, and easy stimulability. On the other hand, in AD, recent memory impairment and disorientation are the main initial symptoms.

The characteristic symptoms are lack of recognition of his disease (insight) from the early stages of the disease. The ability to recognize one's position in a social environment is impaired, that is, the ability to perceive the "self" from a relatively objective standpoint while maintaining subjective awareness (subjective standpoint and self-awareness).

Reading one's own and others' minds (analogizing the movements of one's mind), that is, the ability to read other people's mental states, thoughts and feelings (guess what other people is thinking), impairment of social interpersonal behavior, impairment of self-behavioral control, and blunted affect, and lack of awareness of disease, etc. are impaired. This "theory of mind" is impaired in FTLD compared to AD.

Although there are complaints about the language disorder itself, perception of the disease with a sense of seriousness has been lost and the impact of speech disturbance on the daily life is diluted.

Concerning emotional change they are euphoric, but

there are also cases where they are very impatient and sullen. Emotional dullness and expressionless face are often seen. In addition, some FTLDs have a cold, incommunicable precoxic feeling, such as one received from a schizophrenic patient.

Precoxic feeling is a kind of indescribable peculiar feeling seen in schizophrenia, along with hardness of facial expression, coldness, awkwardness of attitude, lack of emotional communication, strange abruptness, etc. It is a comprehensive feeling intuitively grasped from the frequently encountered personality of a schizophrenia. Euphoric, child-playing personality changes (moria) are indicated by disorders of the orbital plane of the frontal lobe.

Increased distractibility is sometimes observed, that is, interest shifts to novel stimuli one after another.

Complementary phenomenon is observed. When the first half of a proverb is said, the second half is said even when instructed not to say it (strongly restrained)(above mentioned).

The patients immediately begin to sing a song, lured by some word and air.

Compulsive reading: Read out the characters on the sign board that come into sight.

Compulsive verbal response: When an object or examiner's actions are presented during an examination, the patient compulsively responds verbally though he is instructed not to react. (When a person shows a scissors-shaped hand, it is verbalized as "scissors", "V" or "2"). Like echolanguage and echoact, they often respond in the same manner as the stimuli, but in compulsive verbal responses, they are verbally able to respond to the stimuli of actions and objects, and in compulsive reading, they are able to read aloud to letter stimuli.

Echo language is sometimes seen such as "How are you?" →"I'm fine."

Antisocial or instinctive behavior such as "going my own way" caused by disinhibition due to disturbance of the orbital surface of the frontal lobe or association with the temporal lobe is the result of disengagement of inhibition from the anterior association area against the limbic system.

He habitually shoplifts the candies that are lined up in the store without hesitation.

Lack of thinking (lazy thinking), no seriousness is shown in the approach to testing, and he answers arbitrarily or hums a melody during the examination.

The patient walks out of the doctor's office or examination room willfully when he loses interest (walk-away behavior).

He shows lack of sociality absolutely, no consideration for social relationships or surroundings, no signs of embarrassment even when mistakes are pointed out (the patient himself has no ill intentions), and is open-minded.

Stereotypic behavior (stereotypy) is observed in almost all cases, caused by disorder of the orbital surface of the frontal lobe and also the temporal lobe. This is thought to be the result of derestriction from the anterior association area to the basal ganglia. It is also an important symptom for differentiation from AD. On the ward, stereotypic behavior is sitting in a fixed chair in the day room. Stereotypic roaming is seen in everyday life. They keep walking the same course of several kilometers all day long, or go around the course of several kilometers every day, committing petty crimes such as money thieves and stealing flowers and fruits along the way. Stereotypic eating behavior disorder that sticks to a small number of fixed foods and dishes, and stereotyped cooking in women, reducing the variety of side dishes to make are characteristics are frequently observed and miso soup ingredients do not change. Stereotypic behavior is strongly time-regulated and obsessive-compulsive (time-scheduled life). During medical examinations, patients frequently look at their watches and pay attention to the time. His behaviors are regulated on the time axis, not only minutes and hours, but also days and weeks, and actions are regulated by the days of the week.

Music box clock symptom appears in the form of talking about the same content in a group.

Obsessive compulsive symptoms may be seen such as obsessive compulsive checking to lock the door, washing hands, and compulsive/ceremonial behavior such as counting the numbers when going up the stairs and stepping back after a few steps. Obsessive-compulsive symptoms are commonly associated with the lower part of prefrontal cortex, precingulate gyrus, and striatal regions.

Repetitive behavior such as constant rubbing or crackling of hands on knees are seen. Linguistically, it appears in the form of tautology and repetitive writing.

Guiraud summarized as PEMA syndrome (repetitive

verbal palilalie, reverberant verbal echolalie, mutisme, amimie) are observed, associated with dysfunction of the striatum (Guiraud P: Encephale 31:229, 1936). PES syndrome (repetitive language, palilalie/echolingual language/stereotypic behavior) summarized by Tissot (Tissot R: La Maladie de Pick. Paris: Masson et al, 1975) is associated with the frontal convexity atrophy and the temporal lobe atrophy.

Due to dysfunction of the medial frontal lobe, the anterior cingulate gyrus, and the frontal lobe convexity, spontaneity is reduced. VD's decline of spontaneity is often seen, but in contrast to FTLD's decline of spontaneity, FTLD coexists with stereotypic behavior and restlessness in the early stage of the disease, and stereotypic behavior occurs when he is napping. Suddenly he starts stereotypic roaming. This is different from the spontaneous decline in VD, where the patient stays still in the same place all day long without being spoken to.

When asked a question, he does not give a serious answer and immediately answers "I don't know." In general, spontaneity decline is said to be related to disorders of the medial surface of the frontal lobe, especially the anterior cingulate gyrus, but it is also related to atrophy of the frontal lobe convexity.

The patients come up with one creative idea after another, but lack the attention and concentration which is necessary to actually carry it out, and their interest quickly shifts to other ideas (increased distractibility).

Eating behavior disorder is caused by frontal orbital surface and insular gyrus disorder. The incidence of eating behavior disorder is very high compared to AD. Changes in appetite, tastes, and eating habits are observed: especially in the early stages, increased appetite, eating a lot of sweets such as chocolate and juice. Swallowing without chewing thoroughly and eating faster are also observed.

He sticks to a fewer item of food. It is due to disturbance of the neural circuit over the orbital surface of the frontal lobe and the insular gyrus (stereotyped eating behavior).

The executive function is disturbed, and the process becomes short-sighted, reflexive, standardized, and unreflective. It becomes repetitive, stereotyped, and reverberant due to reflexive processing based on impaired insight of his mental condition, increased susceptibility, and disinhibition. Increased distractibility (difficulty of maintaining attention) and reduced mobility are associated in all these processes.

MND type FTLD

In the MND type, ALS is frequently encountered in addition to the behavioral abnormalities and mental symptoms of FTLD. Therefore, the symptoms of ALS are striking such as dysphagia caused by bulbar palsy, muscle atrophy of upper extremity, muscle fasciculation. However, the muscle strength of the lower extremities is preserved and walking is often possible. Primitive reflexes such as grasping, sucking, and palpating are observed in the middle to late stages. It progresses rapidly and has a poor prognosis.

§34 Increased Influence/Environmental dependency syndrome

Environmental dependency syndrome was first reported in his case and proposed by Lhermitte (Lhermitte F, et al: Ann Neurol 19: 335, 1986). The causal lesion is antero~inferior part of the frontal lobe~head of the caudate nucleus. The symptom is results of damage of the anterior association area, loss of control over the posterior association area, and release of the situational dependence inherent in the posterior association area. The threshold by the stimulus from the outside and the inner requirement has been lowered, and the processing has become short-circuited, reflexive, and non-reflecting.

When a patient is led to a certain environment, he behaves in accordance with the environment as if he was commanded by that environment, that is, increased susceptibility. When you take a patient into an apartment, say it is a museum, and when the patient is ruled by the word (induced type), he finds a picture that's been removed from the wall and placed underneath, and he nails it to the wall. There is also an incidental type that appears accidentally in everyday life.

Placing a toothbrush in front of them starts brushing their teeth (utilization behavior). If you show your gloves, he wears them. He will use the pencils, scissors, combs, etc. that are in front of him because he will be eager to use.

To imitate and reproduce the examiner's behavior (pantomime of customary actions in daily life such as "akanbe," "come on," "goodbye," etc.) (imitation behavior). In daily life, when the caregiver tilts his head, the patient responds by echoing or mimicking the caregiver's words (echo language) or action (imitation action).

To summarize the diagnosis of FTLD

1. A history of insidious onset and slowly progressive decline in work capacity for at least 6 months.
2. Impairment of social and interpersonal behavior are already observed in the early stage, that is, anti-social, disinhibitory speech and behavior, abnormal sexual behavior, poor manners, lack of social elegance and decorum.
3. Impaired control of self-behavior from an early age, that is, low motivation, lethargy, hyperactivity, restlessness, roaming, deviations from conventional behavior.
4. Emotional blunting from an early stage, which denotes indifference and inappropriate emotional shallowness with lack of emotional kindness, empathy, consideration for others, and even lack of concern for others.
5. Lack of early awareness of disease is frequently observed from the early stage. It is defined as a lack of awareness of psychiatric symptoms or apathy regarding the social, occupational, and economic consequences of mental dysfunction. It is a symptom that is commonly recognized when dementia progresses, but it is characterized by frequently being conspicuous from the early stage in FTLD.

Miscellaneous phenomenon in dementia

§35 Why are the patients with dementia wandering?

When the patients started wandering, he had a purpose, but lately he has forgotten it because of his memory disturbance. Sometimes he goes out at an unbelievable time due to his lack of awareness of time. Due to impaired spatial awareness, it is impossible to return from where he arrived. He doesn't recognize the feeling of fatigue, so he goes far. Sometimes wandering is explained like this (maybe it should be understood like this).

Wandering is also said to be common in AD and the causative foci are often associated with the right precuneus. It is observed when the ability to walk is preserved, and becomes incapable when physical ability decreases. In our ward a patient (a former English teacher) was constantly wandering around the ward, so when I asked him "Why are you wandering?" He replied with a sense of humor "I am looking for peace."

Dementia and olfactory impairment

In general, Parkinson's disease is most likely to cause olfactory disturbance (75% of PD) although most patients with Parkinson's disease don't become aware of olfactory disturbance (Sengoku R, et al: Automatic Nervous System 58: 294, 2021). Dementia patients also often present with olfactory impairment.

Among dementia diseases, AD is the most likely to cause olfactory disturbance due to deposition of amyloid in the olfactory epithelium and olfactory bulb (Sakai M, et al: Jap J Neuropsychol 33:167, 2017).

Incidentally, the olfactory pathway differs from other sensory system. The information is sent directly to the limbic system without going through the thalamus (olfactory epithelium of the nasal cavity → olfactory tubercle → amygdala, piriform cortex → olfactory inner cortex → hippocampus and orbital frontal lobe, where α-synuclein protein is likely to accumulate).

Dementia and gustatory disorder

Gustatory disorders are also common in dementia. We don't really know why dementia often presents with taste disorders, but it has been said empirically that people with dementia have a strong tendency to prefer sweets. It is assumed that regression (anxiety from frustration, escape, etc.) and behavior seeking pleasant stimulation are related. Carbohydrates are mild drugs (on the other hand, narcotics are hard drugs), which cause regressing of anxiety from frustration, and he feels release and escape from stress by an increase in dopamine secretion, and then he seeks pleasant stimulus further (even normal people have dependencies!). Potato chips, chocolate, hamburgers, donuts, cakes, cola, and cider have similar effects. In Japan, one in five people has this dependence.

Clinical study in patients with AD show that the threshold for all tastes (sweet, salty, sour, and bitter) is elevated, with sweet being the highest, followed by sour (Sakai M, et al : Jap J Neuropsychol 33:167, 2017). In AD, self-restraint is difficult against dependence, so is it possible that sweet tastes are sought more?

As a side note, the gustatory sensation is transmitted by a complex pathway for neurotransmission : taste buds, chorda tympani nerve, glossopharyngeal nerve, superior laryngeal nerve, great superficial pyramidal nerve → nucleus of the medulla oblongata solitarius → thalamus → island, frontal valve lid part (primary gustatory area) →orbital part of frontal lobe, amygdala (secondary gustatory cortex) → hypothalamus. Because the conduction pathways of smell and taste intersect (because of the adverse electrical and anatomical consequences of impaired pathways), is it possible that patients with olfactory disorders are more likely to develop dysgeusia (Matters RD, et al: J Am Diet Assoc 94: 50, 1994) (De Jong N, et al: J Gerontol A Biol Sci Med Sci: 54: B324, 1999) ?

§36 Why are people with dementia prone to weight loss?

In the first place, even if there is no dementia, people with abnormal sense of smell and taste may feel that food is not delicious and may experience a decrease in appetite and decrease of digestive juice, leading to weight loss and malnutrition. BPSD in dementia sometimes presents with overeating, but mostly weight loss. Why do dementia patients often lose weight? There are many papers but there are no conclusive papers. From the point of view of family medicine, when the sense of smell and taste decreases (regardless of the recovery period, regardless of whether dementia is present or not), the stimulation from these senses decreases, and the food tastes bad, leading to a loss of appetite. Even if the entire meal is consumed (unless the meal is delicious and pleasant to eat), digestive function decline (decreased secretion of saliva and digestive juices, and decreased motility of the digestive tract) may occur, resulting in nutritional deficiencies followed by weight loss.

A paper from academic societies related to weight loss and dementia is described about a relationship between AD, MMSE and weight loss though it is an observational study and not a decisive scientific paper (Soto ME, et al: J Alzheimer Dis 28: 647, 2012). Weight loss occurs in 70% of patients with dementia (Morris CH, et al :Br J Psychiatry.154:801,1989). In addition, weight loss has been reported to precede the diagnosis of dementia (Barnett-Connor E, et al: J Am Geriatr Soc 44:1147,1996).

The mechanisms of losing weight in convalescent rehabilitation are described in due order.

1. A stress state occurs according to the severity of the disease in the acute phase.
2. Production of stress hormones (glucocorticoids, noradrenaline) and inflammatory cytokines (TNF-α, IL-1β, IL-6) (Chamorro A, et al: Stroke 38:1097, 2007).
3. Stress generates endogenous energy.
4. If this continues without disappearing not only in the acute phase but also in the recovery phase, the problem of losing weight appears. There are quite a few cases in which the stress state of the acute phase persists even in the recovery phase. That may be CARS, and the problem of endogenous energy continues.
5. That is, considering the excessively generated endogenous energy (if the initial disease is severe), the policy of underfeeding is implicit in the acute phase as an empirical methods derived from clinician's experience in patient management. There has been some consensus on these nutritional issues among intensive care societies, emergency medicine societies, neurosurgery societies, and surgical societies. The clinician comes to deeply understand with his sore spot. Consensus has been obtained on this issue, which has been clinically accepted (Hitotsumatsu T, et al: Jpn J Stroke 39: 177, 2017). The above mechanism has also been confirmed in translational research (Terashima H, et al : J Jap Soc Intensive Care Med 20:359, 2013). Incidentally, it is an established theory that immune function is inversely correlated with the severity of stroke in the acute phase of stroke (this is called stroke induced immuno-depression) (Chamorro A, et al : Nat Rev Neurol 8:401, 2012).
6. It may be a little sidetracking, but I would like to talk about mechanism of immunosuppression in stroke because it is a very important matter. Since stroke patients in my wards account for more than 70%, but not all, I have created this section for the purpose of your under-

standing and reference.

① Inflammatory cytokines (TNF-α, IL-1β, IL-6) are produced from damaged brain lesions and trigger the hypothalamic-pituitary-adrenal cortical system and sympathetic nervous system (resulting in excess secretion of glucocorticoids and noradrenaline) (Prass K, et al : J Exp Med 198:725, 2003).

② The enhancement of the above-mentioned system causes a decrease in MHC class II molecules, a decrease in the number of circulating immune cells and lymphocytes, resulting in a decrease in immunity. As a result of these, what happens next is the living body's defense reaction to suppress the excessive function of the system mentioned above. That is, CARS is induced to control the activation of the above-mentioned system. The high incidence of pneumonia after stroke is related not only to dysphagia and disturbed consciousness, but also to this weakened immune system.

7. In this state, if excess nutrition (exogenous energy) is given (even if calculated by the Harris-Benedict formula and taking into account the physical activity level), metabolic adverse events occur (because of overfeeding). It is glucose toxicity and nutritional stress due to glucose overload.

8. Regarding glucose toxicity, oxidative stress due to excess production of active oxygen due to glucose overload, and among the oxidative stress especially mitochondrial stress is important. Mitochondrial stress is caused by mitochondrial inner membrane hyperpermeability and opening of mitochondrial PTP, followed by mitochondrial dysfunction. This also contributes to individual cell injury (exacerbating the course of the disease).

9. Even if insulin is administered to treat hyperglycemia (during glucose toxicity) and blood glucose levels are corrected, it is taken up into skeletal muscle cells and excessively renews glucose metabolism, causing overproduction of ROS and oxidative stress. In addition, due to an increase in the total secretion amount of insulin in the body, the secretion of noradrenaline also increases and muscle protein breakdown occurs, making it difficult to improve the situation and only exacerbating it.

10. Excessive noradrenaline promotes the breakdown of body fat and glycogen (because noradrenaline correlates with insulin secretion) and supplies fatty acids and glucose, and it converts to synthesis (recycling). However, under the condition of overfeeding it consumes energy during synthesis, so it is called a futile cycle, which eventually increases resting energy expenditure (REE) (Terashima H, et al : J Jap Soc Intensive Care Med 20:359, 2013).

11. Even impairment due to glucose toxicity alone is fatal, but apart from that, protein impairment also causes nutritional stress and induces cell damage, the main of which is the impairment (suppression) of autophagy (Terashima H, et al : J Jap Soc Intensive Care Med 20:359, 2013).

12. In other words, normally, infectious substances such as extracellular bacteria and surplus biopolymer components are taken into the cell by endocytosis (the mechanism by which the cell takes in extracellular substances by endosomes), and this is captured inside the phagosome (cytoplasmic vesicle). Some useful substances are absorbed into cells and reused. Vesicles surrounding unnecessary molecules and intracellular unnecessary components that have not been reused (objects to be digested when autophagy autolyzes intracellular organelles, etc. in autophagosomes) fuse and coalesce with lysosomes (in lysosomes it has degradative enzymes), it decomposes internal waste products and kills pathogens (Fig.13).

13. The remaining are released outside the cell as exosomes (50-150 nm) (extracellular vesicles) and carry out intercellular information transmission and protein

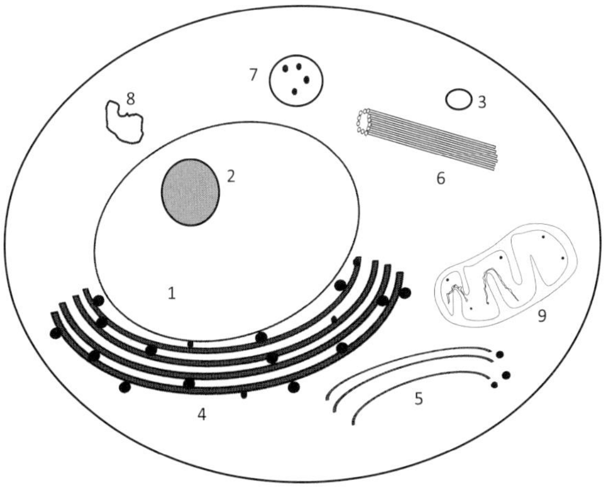

Fig.13. Schematic drawing of cross section of a cell: (1) nucleus, (2) nucleolus, (3) ribosome, (4) rough endoplasmic reticulum, (5) Golgi apparatus, (6) microtubules, (7) centriole, (8) lysosome, (9) mitochondrion.

transport.

14. There are MHC molecules on the surface of exosomes, which are very important molecules for immunity (pathogens taken in by dendritic cells or B cells are decomposed into peptides, bound to MHC class II or class I molecules, which is presented on the surface and presented to naive killer T cells or helper T cells. This is the beginning of innate immunity to acquired immunity). In addition to immune function, exosomes protect neurons from oxidative stress and promote the degradation of amyloid β. This mechanism is also impaired.

15. The autophagic mechanism described in 11-14 is disturbed by overfeeding, followed by promoting infection (lowering immunity), damage to the repair system of cell damage, various disorders at the cell level, and furthermore, dysfunction and delayed recovery at the organ level. Incidentally, glucose, amino acids, and insulin are potent inhibitors against autophagy.

16. The possibility of malnutrition and loss of skeletal muscle due to post-ICU treatment syndrome (PICS) cannot be ignored (Sato N, et al: Intensivist 10,153, 2018).

17. Muscle breakdown becomes more pronounced as the number of failing organs increases.

18. Incidentally, with age, a substance called "rubicon" is produced that reduces autophagy, which leads to progression of ageing phenomenon of the elderly (Imoto H, et al: Cell Reports 38, 110444, 2022), and may also be involved in weight loss in elderly patients.

Specifically, half of the patients after the treatment in ICU admitted to convalescent rehabilitation ward show ICU-acquired weakness. They need rehabilitation but cannot do adequately for diarrhea, hyperglycemia, arrhythmia and delirium, which are induced by metabolic abnormality probably associated with cytokine storm, etc. In the ICU and convalescent rehabilitation ward, nutritional management is necessary. In the convalescent rehabilitation CARS is still lasting in not a few patients whose diseases are not cured, or have complication. For these cases, the same nutritional management done in the ICU is also necessary to be continued in the convalescent rehabilitation ward depending on the severity.

For the treatment oral intake is the basic policy, and enteral nutrition using a nasogastric tube is started without a waiting period even in cases of difficulty in oral intake due to disturbance of consciousness or dysphagia. Standard protocol (Std) as a protocol for enteral nutrition; 80% of basal energy expenditure (BEE) is satisfied 4-5 days after starting nutrition. Permissive under (Und); 600Kcal/day for the first 7 days. Trophic (Trp); 400Kcal/day for the first 5 days, depending on the severity. Std was applied for mild cases, Und for moderate cases, and Trp for highly invasive cases with ventilator management or after surgical treatment. Std needs to continue until CARS disappears.

In summary, a variety of factors can contribute to weight loss during convalescent rehabilitation. The most serious of these is that the poor course of the underlying disease often results in an unavoidable increase in endogenous energy, and the administration of exogenous energy (even though it is not considered excessive) ultimately exceeds REE. This overfeeding causes metabolic disorders such as glucose toxicity and nutritional stress, resulting in mitochondrial disorders, apoptosis, suppression of autophagy, immunodeficiency, delayed repair of cell damage, skeletal muscle metabolic disorders, muscle proteolysis, etc.

Why do dementia patients in convalescent rehabilitation often lose weight?

Why do dementia patients in convalescent rehabilitation often lose weight? It is true that dementia patients in convalescent rehabilitation often lose weight. In our ward of convalescent rehabilitation department 70% of the dementia patients lose weight while 30% of the non-dementia patients do. The reason of losing weight of dementia patients in convalescent rehabilitation are appetite loss caused by decrease of olfactory and gustatory sense, progression of dementia, decrease of degraded amyloid β derived by the autophagy disorder, production of rubicon which disturbs autophagy, the countless harmful factors mentioned in the previous section, etc. It is not difficult to imagine that dementia patients probably have more of these adverse factors. It is very complicated because the causes of weight loss in dementia patients overlap with the causes of weight loss due to the burden of convalescent rehabilitation.

§37 Post-intensive care syndrome (PICS)

PICS occurs in 30-80% of patients during ICU stay or within 5 years after discharge. It occurs after the treatment of severe disease: for instance, motor dysfunction (it is called ICU-acquired weakness. It is polyneuropathy with axon injury resulting in extremity muscle weakness and sensory disturbance) (Bolton CF, et al: J Neurol Neurosurg Psychiatry 47:1223.1984), psychiatric disorders (depression, PTSD, cephalosporin-induced antibiotic-associated encephalopathy), and cognitive dysfunction (delirium, language and memory disorders, and hippocampal atrophy).

Concerning the causes and triggers, it occurs in 33% after mechanical ventilation and 50% after sepsis. Depressive state, MOF, PTSD, low education level, alcohol dependence, ARDS, abnormal blood sugar levels, sedatives, steroids, muscle relaxants, aminoglycoside antibiotics (causes muscle weakness in the extremities), etc. may be associated with the outbreak of PICS. Prevention is needed through early rehabilitation.

Symptoms occur not only in the individual but also in the family which is called post-intensive care syndrome-family (PICS-F), and have long-term effects (Davidson LE, et al: Crit Care Med 40: 618, 2012). The symptoms are psychological symptom such as anxiety, depression, PTSD, sleep disturbance, disturbance of attention.

Lastly, this chapter has come to an end, but there are still many other dementias, which are caused by prion disease, hypothyroidism, normal pressure hydrocephalus, herpes encephalitis, chronic alcoholism, vitamin B12 deficiency, etc. Unfortunately, I can't describe it any more due to space constraints.

Chapter 3 Clinical stroke

This chapter briefly describes the minimum basic clinical matters necessary for rehabilitation physicians regarding recent trends in stroke. You are able to read books and papers for details about each disease.

§1 Epidemiology and pathogenesis of stroke (general knowledge)

As is a well-known fact, the epidemiology and pathogenesis of stroke will be briefly summarized in this section. There are 1.2 million cases of stroke each year. It is the 4th leading cause of death, and the number of deaths is gradually decreasing. The three major types of the disease are cerebral hemorrhage, cerebral infarction, and subarachnoid hemorrhage. 40% of bedridden patients are due to stroke, and the average length of hospital stay is the highest among all diseases. Currently, 62.7% of strokes are cerebral infarctions and 23.0% are cerebral hemorrhages, and although the incidence of cerebral hemorrhages has decreased considerably in Japan, compared to Europe and the United States, the rate of cerebral hemorrhages is higher. In Japan, the mortality rate for cerebral hemorrhage has fallen below that for cerebral infarction since 1975.

Putaminal hemorrhage often occurs when there is a history of high blood pressure, and patients suddenly experience hemiplegia, impaired consciousness, and speech disorders. Cerebellar hemorrhage manifests as headache, vomiting, and vertigo, and if it progresses, it manifests as consciousness disturbance. Symptoms of subcortical hemorrhage vary depending on the location of the bleeding. Pontine hemorrhage manifests as coma, impaired consciousness, quadriplegia, and respiratory abnormalities, and generally has a poor prognosis. Thalamic hemorrhage causes language impairment and hemiplegia. Cognitive symptoms are somewhat noticeable, and it is more common in the elderly than putaminal hemorrhage. Intracerebral hemorrhage generally occurs due to the rupture of a small aneurysm that occurs in an intracerebral arteriole with a diameter of 200 to 300 μm. In the case of very elderly people, breakdown of the neurovascular unit (blood vessels, vascular endothelial cells, nerve cells, and neuroglial cells work together) can cause intracerebral hemorrhage (particularly in the thalamic hemorrhage). In young people, bleeding occurs due to local damage to blood vessels due to juvenile hypertension. The clinical picture of intracerebral hemorrhage has changed recently. The incidence rate has decreased to the same level as in Europe and the United States, and the proportion of patients with mild symptoms has increased, and this is due to improved management of risk factors and improvements in the living environment. In addition, conservative treatment is increasingly replacing surgery. Furthermore, the onset of disease is no longer related to the season.

Seventy percent of the causes of subarachnoid hemorrhage are rupture of a cerebral aneurysm, which manifests as sudden headache, vomiting, and impaired consciousness. Endovascular surgery is usually the first choice, and the frequency of direct surgery is decreasing year by year. Doctors, who are said to be "the hands of God," are becoming less and less active in the field of apoplexy.

Lacunar infarctions occur due to occlusion of 0.2 to 0.3 mm arterioles due to degeneration (lipohyalinosis), resulting in infarcts less than 5 mm in size called lacuna (meaning small cavities). In cerebral embolism, a blood clot generates due to cardiac fibrillation, etc., and the embolus that flies from there occludes the blood vessels in the brain. The majority of cerebral embolisms result in hemorrhagic infarction. Symptoms caused by these strokes include local neurological symptoms based on anatomical structure, such as hemiplegia, speech impairment, and dementia. Most cardiogenic cerebral infarctions are caused by atrial fibrillation, which increases with age, but it is often difficult to distinguish between these types of cerebral infarctions. Preventing a patient who has already had a stroke from having another stroke is called secondary prevention. Patients with non-valvular atrial fibrillation are treated with anticoagulants if they have a CHADS2 score of 2 or higher. Factors to consider include congestive heart failure (C), hypertension (H), age 75 years or older (A), diabetes (D), and history of stroke/transient ischemic attack (S2). Since cerebral infarction accounts for as much as 60 to 70% of all strokes, most of the discussion in clinical practice stems from the translational research on molecular biology of cerebral ischemia in Chapter 1.

Metabolic syndrome is based on genetic predisposition, but combined with lifestyle imbalances (overeating, lack of exercise). It causes obesity and insulin resistance. As a result, patients developed glucose intolerance, hypertension, and dyslipidemia. These make cerebrovascular accidents 1.5 to 2 times more likely. The required diagnostic criteria is a waist circumference > 85 cm. The selection items (the following two) are: 1. Neutral fat >150 and/or low HDL cholesterol level <40. 2. Systolic blood pressure >130 and/or diastolic blood pressure >85. 3. Fasting blood sugar >110. By the way, risk factors for cardiovascular disease are: hypertension, smoking, diabetes, abnormal lipid metabolism (hypercholesterolemia, low HDL cholesterolemia <40mg, high LDL cholesterolemia >140mg), obesity (particularly visceral obesity), urinary microalbumin, older age (men >60 years, women >65 years), and family history of early-onset vascular disease. Not surprisingly, the risk factors for stroke are very similar.

Normal blood pressure is below 130/80. The main risk factors for high blood pressure include smoking, excessive salt intake, obesity, excessive alcohol intake, stress, and lack of sleep. Specifically, prevention is: limit salt to less than 6g/day, active intake of vegetables and fruits, limit intake of cholesterol and saturated fatty acids. Maintaining an appropriate weight: BMI (weight [kg]÷[height (m)]^2) of 18 to 25 is normal. Moderate exercise, aimed at people with high blood pressure who do not have cardiovascular disease, should regularly engage in low-intensity aerobic exercise for at least 30 minutes each day. The alcohol limit should be 20-30mL/day for men and 10-20mL/day for women, converted to 100% ethanol. It goes without saying that smoking is prohibited.

The order in which large blood vessels are affected by arteriosclerosis is approximately fixed. The general exacerbation process that leads to the final stage of arteriosclerosis (ultimately leading to cerebral infarction, myocardial infarction, etc.) is: 1. abdominal aorta, iliac artery, 2. coronary artery, 3. femoral artery, popliteal artery, 4. internal carotid artery, 5. vertebrobasilar artery.

There are differences in the progression of vascular lesions between Europe, the United States and Japan. Stenosis of the main intracranial artery is rare in Europe and America, but is common in Japan. The opposite is true for cervical vessels. Moyamoya disease is extremely rare in Europe and America, and is thought to be an Asian disease. Genetic research has confirmed that it started in a person in China 3,000 years ago and spread to the Japanese archipelago as people migrated, and it is said to be an RNF213-related vascular disease based on the susceptibility gene. The diagnostic criteria for Moyamoya disease have changed and now include unilateral disease. Moyamoya like disease (Sato M, et al: Neurosurgery 17:260,1985) is not included in Moyamoya disease (Moyamoya like disease has non-genetic causes).

§2 Treatment

TPA administration in thrombolytic therapy for cerebral infarction can be attempted within 4.5 hours of onset. Drip ship retrieve is a method in which the patient is first administered tPA and then transported to a specialized hospital for clot retrieval therapy, which is recommended.

Mechanical thrombectomy (acute thrombectomy) is widely performed for cerebral infarction, but mechanical thrombectomy for cerebral infarction is now indicated if there is a mismatch area (penumbra) even after 24 hours have passed. Although time from onset is no longer the only issue, mechanical thrombectomy is generally indicated within 16 hours of onset and in cases where the penumbra region is observed. Regarding middle cerebral artery occlusion, occlusions up to M1, and only a few cases more distal than M2 can be indicated and recovered. Preoperatively, the middle cerebral artery region on one side was divided into 10 regions using CT, and the Alberta Stroke Programme Early CT Score (ASPECTS) was evaluated for the presence or absence of early ischemic changes (10 points if no ischemia, 0 points if ischemia is observed over the entire area). The affected area is assessed using MRI, and the extent to which occluded artery was actually recirculated after thrombus retrieval (i.e., effective recanalization rate) is evaluated using the thrombolysis in cerebral infarction (TICI) grade. It is expected that the line will open in one pass. Most neurological findings in acute care hospitals are evaluated by modified Rankin scale, and although FIM assessment is difficult before surgery, there is no evaluation by

FIM even after surgery. It is not clear whether there is any improvement in cognitive function or mental function by the thrombectomy. This will become the first time that several cognitive evaluations including FIM will be performed at a convalescent rehabilitation hospital. Even if the motor disorder improves, significant cognitive dysfunction or mental disorders may remain, which will probably be a major hindrance to reintegration into society or daily life, but staff at acute care hospitals rarely notice this. This is similar to the controversy over the surgical timing, techniques, and results of acute cerebral aneurysm craniotomy, in which a simple outcome scale like a modified Rankin scale was previously used. Postoperative evaluation should not be based on it, but I remember that 50 years ago, the above was passionately discussed at academic conferences based on a simple outcome scale. When it comes to surgery, it is not that human hands have become more dexterous or delicate (aside from "God's hands"), but rather that advances in surgical instruments, diagnostic techniques, and preoperative endovascular surgery have improved surgical prognosis and morbidity. Patients admitted to convalescent rehabilitation ward after endovascular surgery sometimes exhibit a variety of conspicuous symptoms. I make the rounds while thinking about why they have developed such symptoms.

The cause of one-quarter of cerebral infarctions is unknown, and this is called an embolic stroke of undetermined source (ESUS). Treatment is difficult, but a study was conducted comparing dabigatran and aspirin, but there was no significant difference between the two (there was no difference in recurrence rate). However, since conventional guidelines recommend antiplatelet drugs, it is recommended to use antiplatelet drugs and then switch to anticoagulant therapy if there is reactivity to anticoagulants in the event of recurrence. Even if ESUS recurs, the cause is still unknown in many cases. However, the incidence of ESUS is said to be reduced to around 5% if thorough scrutiny is conducted.

In arteries where blood flows quickly, primary hemostasis by these platelets forms a thrombus, which is called a white thrombus. Antiplatelet drugs are taken to prevent embolism associated with the white thrombus (non-cardiac cerebral infarction such as atherothrombotic cerebral infarction or lacunar infarction, myocardial infarction, chronic arterial occlusive disease, etc.). Typical drugs that suppress platelet activation include aspirin, clopidogrel, prasugrel, and cilostazol. According to the Stroke Treatment Guidelines 2021, aspirin 160mg to 300mg should be started for early cerebral infarction (within 48 hours) (recommendation level A, evidence level high), or the combination of aspirin and clopidogrel for mild non-cardiogenic cerebral infarction is recommended as a treatment method (recommendation level A, evidence level high) for up to 1 month. Cilostazol 200 mg alone or in combination with aspirin may be considered for the treatment of non-cardiogenic cerebral infarction within 48 hours (recommendation level C, level of evidence: medium). Cilostazol is a phosphodiesterase inhibitor that suppresses the degradation of cyclic AMP and cyclic GMP, which are second messengers in intracellular signal transmission, and has a unique mechanism of action as a drug that positively affects cerebral blood vessels. Unfortunately, it is not as effective as aspirin or clopidogrel (see§10 in chapter Ⅰ).

It is said that the metabolic pathway for clopidogrel is different between Westerners and Japanese people, and there are quite a few cases of poor response to clopidogrel in Asians. Clopidogrel is a prodrug and susceptible to genetic polymorphism (20% of Japanese people are poor metabolizer). Prasugrel is an antiplatelet drug with quick effects. Both clopidogrel and prasugrel are thienopyridine drugs, and their metabolic pathways are different, with clopidogrel mainly using CYP2C19 and prasugrel using CYP3A and CYP2B6 (see§12 in chapter Ⅱ).

Generally, the most commonly used drug is aspirin, and recently it is mostly used in combination with clopidogrel or prasugrel, known as dual antiplatelet therapy (DAPT). DAPT is usually converted to SAPT within one month. After performing a therapy with a flow diverter, DAPT is often used for 3 to 6 months.

In the cardiac field, it is often taken to prevent blood clots in patients undergoing percutaneous coronary intervention (PCI). For heart-related drugs, the basic rule is to reduce to 1 drug within 1 year and use aspirin as a single drug. Regarding cerebral infarction, the upper limit for the combination of the two is 3 months due to the risk of cerebral hemorrhage. Verify now is an instrument that measures the strength of each antiplatelet effect, but there are reports that the measured values should not necessarily be trusted (platelet function is very fragile, and the condition inside the blood vessel may be changed outside the blood vessel easily). As mentioned above, 20% of Japanese people have a low response to clopidogrel, but prasugrel has a relatively rapid effect (it does not need to be measured by Verify now). For drugs other than prasugrel, it is preferable to measure with Verify now (P2Y12 Reaction Unit, PRU) and change drugs.

Anticoagulants inhibit fibrin formation, the final step in blood clot formation (called a red blood clot because fibrin engulfs red blood cells). Anticoagulants are mainly taken to prevent cardiogenic cerebral embolism caused by large and strong blood clots. Among anticoagulants, the representative drugs are warfarin, the thrombin inhibitor dabigatran (the antagonist is idarucizumab), and the three Xa inhibitors: rivaroxaban, apixaban, and edoxaban (the reversal drug is andexanet alfa). All drugs other than warfarin used to be called NOACs (novel anticoagulants), but recently they are called DOACs (direct oral anticoagulants). Very simply, antiplatelet drugs are used for non-cardiac embolism, and anticoagulants are used for cardiogenic cerebral embolism. Anticoagulants should never be used together. However, it is not uncommon for antiplatelet drugs and anticoagulants to be used together. Anticoagulant therapy after mechanical valve replacement is indicated only for warfarin, not DOAC. DOAC is contraindicated for severe renal impairment. DOAC should be started on the 1st day for TIA, on the 2nd day for mild ischemia, on the 3rd day for moderate ischemia, and on the 4th day for severe ischemia; 1-2-3-4 day rule is the general international standard, but in Japan, administration began a little earlier than this standard.

The number one cause of cerebral embolism is atrial fibrillation, and it is said that approximately 90% of the locations where blood clots form are in the "left atrial appendage" located in the left atrium. Percutaneous left atrial appendage closure is a treatment method that involves inserting a device called Watchman into the left atrial appendage using a catheter through a vein in the groin and closing it to prevent the outflow of blood clots caused by atrial fibrillation, thereby preventing cerebral embolism.

Endovascular surgery is widely performed for cerebral aneurysms, and this field is further developing. New devices have been developed to treat large aneurysms that could not be treated with clipping or conventional endovascular surgery, or aneurysms in areas that were difficult to reach. These include stent assist therapy and flow diverter, the latter of which include Pipeline, FRED, and Surpass. The aneurysm with a maximum diameter of 10 mm or more, and wide neck (neck length of 4 mm or more, or with a dome/neck ratio of less than 2) has been treated by endovascular therapy. Currently, flow diverters are also being used in the vertebrobasilar artery system. These Pipeline, FRED, Lvis, and Surpass are devices for treating cerebral aneurysms that provide new treatment options for large and giant cerebral aneurysms. Furthermore, the new Pulse Rider is a metal system that prevents the coil from prolapse from the neck filled in the bifurcation aneurysm, and is a new device that reduces the amount of metal in the stent placed in the pipeline. Further progress is expected in these endovascular treatments. However, we also need to be careful about new complications associated with this.

§3 Miscellaneous events after stroke treatment

Once the clinical course has stabilized to some extent, post-operative rehabilitation is performed from the acute stage or mainly during the recovery stage. Constraint-induced movement therapy (CI therapy) is one of the best for upper limb rehabilitation. Rehabilitation robots are being introduced, and they are considered to be significantly effective in helping walking independently. Welwalk (manufactured by Fujita Health University and Toyota), Locomat, HAL, and Reogo (upper limb rehabilitation robots, available in exoskeleton and end effector types). Other treatments include IVES treatment, magnetic resonance stimulation, and rTMS, which is thought to be an extension of the conventional psychiatric electroconvulsive therapy (ECT), but the mechanism of action is not very well understood, just like ECT. Molecular biological regeneration of nerve cells includes methods mediated by cytokines, methods aimed at rebuilding neural circuits through IPS cells, organoids, etc. These are treatments for penumbra (see Chapter Ⅰ).

Epilepsy is common after a stroke (Galovic M, et al: Lancet 17:143, 2018) (Haapaniemi E, et al: Stroke

45:1971, 2014). Epilepsy is most common in children and young adults. In people aged 65 and over, it increases with age. Among elderly patients, cerebrovascular causes account for 30% to 40%, which is the most common cause, and AD related causes are the second most common. The cause is unknown, accounting for 20-30%, which is also a large number. Unlike convulsions in young people, half of the seizures are non-lesional late onset epilepsy or non-convulsive epilepsy, which is a characteristic of epilepsy in the elderly.

§4 Stroke and immunity

There are many reports regarding relation between stroke and immunity. The cell death and subsequent inflammatory processes caused by stroke not only exacerbate neurological deficits and trigger local inflammatory immune responses in the brain, but also alter systemic immunity, leading to immunosuppression and infection (mainly pneumonia and urinary tract infections). It can lead to a decrease in the number of immune cells in the circulation, increasing the risk of infection. This causes a decrease in the expression of MHC class Ⅱ molecule, leading to increased susceptibility to bacterial infections (Vogelgesang A, et al: Stroke 39: 237, 2008).

Activation of adrenergic nerves is caused, leading to catecholamine secretion and triggering immunosuppressive mechanisms after stroke (Wong CH, et al: Science 334:101, 2011). Experimentally and clinically, it has been reported that catecholamine blood levels increase after stroke, and lymphopenia also appears (Liesz A, et al: PloS One 8:8, e74839, 2013) (Chamorro A, et al: Stroke 40:1262, 2009). Catecholamines act through β-adrenergic receptors on immune cells, decreasing TNF-α and increasing IL-10. Use of β-adrenergic receptor antagonists (β-blockers) in post-stroke mice reduces bacterial complication and mortality, suggesting a serious adverse drug reaction of catecholamines in post-stroke immunosuppression (Konstantin P, et al: J Exp Med 198:725, 2003).

After stroke, cells in the area of necrosis release HMGB1 causing an immunosuppressive state during the subacute phase of stroke leading to pneumonia (Walter U, et al: J Neurol 254:1323, 2007). Furthermore, TLR-2, TLR-4, and RAGE are expressed on many cells and mediate the inflammatory effects of HMGB1 through activation of NF-κB. The high incidence of pneumonia in post-stroke patients is not only due to dysphagia and impaired consciousness, but also changes in the immune system are said to be involved in the pathogenesis of stroke-related pneumonia. Many stroke patients have swallowing dysfunction, which may be related to inappropriate dopamine transmission, and D1 dopamine receptor blockade has been reported to inhibit the swallowing reflex and reduce substance P secretion (Jia YX et al: Am J Physiol 274:R76, 1998). It has also been observed that elderly patients with aspiration pneumonia have lower sputum levels of substance P, which is involved in coughing and swallowing reflexes. Elevated serum levels of substance P after treatment with angiotensin-converting enzyme inhibitors are associated with decreased aspiration (Arai T, et al: Neurology 61:1625, 2003). The oral microbiota also changes rapidly after stroke, and colonization by Gram-negative bacteria occurs more frequently than in non-stroke patients (Millms B, et al: Gerontology 49:173, 2003). Bacterial species including Streptococcus pneumoniae, Pseudomonas aeruginosa, Escherichia coli, and Enterobacter cloacae have been isolated and identified (Yan L, et al: Cell Biochem Biophys 71:731, 2015). As perspective therapies, experimental studies have shown that treatments that block beta-adrenergic receptors reduce infections after stroke (Prass K, et al: J Exp Med 198:725,2003) . Similarly, poststroke patients treated with beta-blockers have been reported to have a lower incidence of pneumonia and significantly reduced 30-day mortality than patients not receiving beta-blockers (Dziedzic T, et al: J Neurol Sci 252:53, 2007). In conclusion a local inflammatory immune response in the brain, alters systemic immunity, leading to immunosuppression and susceptibility to infections (mainly pneumonia and urinary tract infections). Hyperactivation of β-adrenergic stimulation and cholinergic anti-inflammatory pathways are involved in immune dysfunction following acute stroke (Westendorp W, et al: BMC Neurol 11:110, 2011) (Chamorro A, et al: Stroke 38:1097, 2007).

Chapter 4 Novel coronavirus infection

§1 Pathophysiology

Covid 19 is slowly waning in 2024, but many hospitals and healthcare facilities are still on alert. However, there is no doubt that it is an infectious disease that can lead to death in some cases, so let's take another look at the problems with Covid 19. First, I would like to share some common knowledge about the novel coronavirus infection (covid 19).

1. There are three possible routes of infection, all of which are possible. It has been five years since covid 19 outbreak occurred, and I am revisiting the route of infection every day as I make my rounds.
   ① Droplet transmission: Size of droplet is 5μm or more and included in such as cough, sputum, saliva. Infection range is 2m diameter
   ② Contact infection: Virus lives shorter on the copper surface, but it still lives for about 6 hours. It lives longer on the other surface.
   ③ Droplet nuclei infection, airborne infection, aerial infection: Viruses survive in the air as an aerosol due to coughing and sneezing for 3 hours. Mycobacterium tuberculosis is 2-4μ, so it is similar to infection with tuberculosis.
2. Basic reproduction number: Infection spreads one person to how many people. Corona is 1.4-2.5, tentatively 2.2, the same as influenza. Measles is 12-18.
3. The accuracy of the PCR test is not high (around 70%). There are other LAMP methods, NEAR method, and antigen tests, but they are lower than this.
4. Antibody tests are only considered as reference values (Antibody levels may not rise even if infected. It is difficult to determine at what level immunity has been acquired. Antibody levels may also rise in other viral infections) .
5. The entry site of the virus is the site of the angiotensin converting enzyme receptor 2 (ACE2). Many ACE2 receptors exist in alveolar type II cells, vascular endothelial cells, heart, kidney, testis, intestinal tract, and retina (causing retinal microangiopathy and scotoma).
6. Case fatality rate (CFR): 2.3% , but if the patients are over 80 years old, CFR is 14.8%, and they have cardiovascular complications 10.5%, DM 7.3%, hypertension 6%, cancer 5.3%, chronic lung disease 6.3%.
7. Severe covid 19 in young people may be caused by TLR7 mutation, Type 1, 2, IFN response decline, etc.
8. Blood draw results from severe covid 19 patients are as follows. ① troponin ↑ (20% of patients)due to cardiac disorder, ② due to viral infection, lymphocytes↑, LDH↑, ③ due to DIC, abnormal coagulation, D-dimer↑, mild thrombocytopenia, ④ cytokine impairment leads to IL-6↑, ⑤ pulmonary interstitial injury leads to KL-6↑.
9. Antibody dependent enhancement (ADE) issue.
10. In the first place, mild viral infections should be cured by innate immunity, and even severe ones should be cured by the adaptive immune system, but covid 19 is often not easily resolved like this.
11. A graph showing the clinical course of the original Wuhan strain type before covid 19 was mutated (Fig 14).

§2 Innate and acquired immunity mechanisms

I would like to briefly describe the phenomena that occur when this virus invades the body. First, the pathogen-recognizing sensor on the membrane of the intracellular vesicle endosome inside the macrophage is activated. It begins when certain pattern recognition receptors, such as toll-like receptors (TLR 3, 7, 9, etc.), recognize viral RNA. This is how the virus enters the cell.

In this way; when macrophages eat viruses as natural immunity, macrophages are activated and secrete many cytokines, among which chemokines play the biggest role, and chemokines call for the help of other macrophages. Neutrophils also rush to support. Lymph nodes have a T-cell area (paracortex) and a B-cell area (cortex). T cells in the lymph node secrete the chemokines CCL19 and CCL21. T cell accumulation expressing chemokine receptor 7 (CCR7) is promoted (that is, CCL19 and CCL21 are ligands for CCR7). Incidentally, CCR7 is a G protein-coupled receptor in signal transduction. The chemokine CXCL13 expresses in the B-cell area of lymph nodes and attracts CXCR5-expressing B cells.

Around the same time, acquired immunity is activated, and dendritic cells take up the virus, activate it, and de-

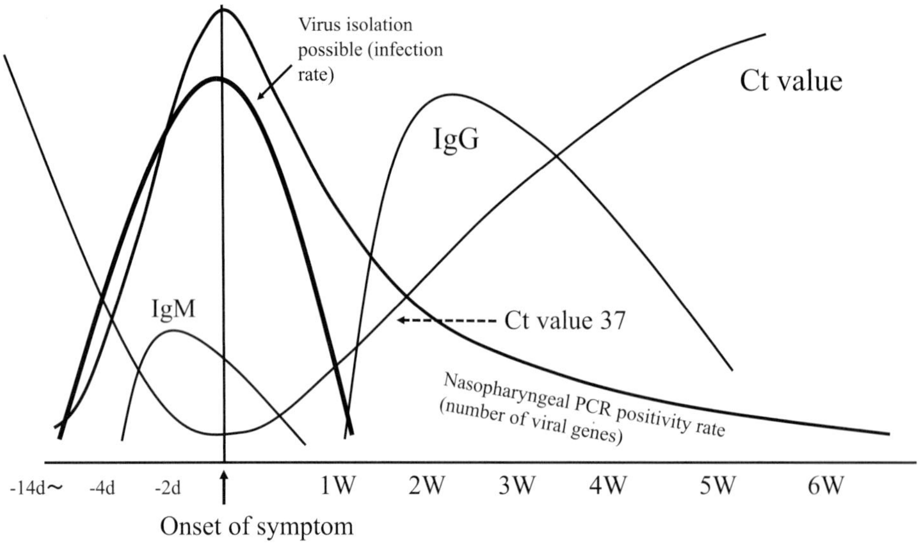

Fig.14. Schematized graph showing time course of covid 19.
The time before the onset of symptom may vary somewhat depending on the presence or absence of ADE, etc.

grade it into peptides, presenting a complex of MHC class II molecules + viral degradation products to naive helper T cells. Naive helper T cells are activated to become activated helper T cells. There are two types of T cells (T lymphocytes): helper T cells (CD4-positive T cells) that express CD4 molecules on the cell surface, and killer T cells (CD8-positive T cells) that express CD8 molecules. MHC class II molecules need to bind to CD4, and MHC class 1 molecules need to bind to CD8 to activate each cell.

Dendritic cells present antigens on MHC1 molecules and their counterparts are naive killer T cells. Therefore, dendritic cells have both MHC I and II molecules, and activated helper T cells and nerve killer T cells stick to each.

The antigen adheres to the B cell antigen recognition receptor of naive B cells, is ingested and decomposed into peptides, is presented to MHC class II molecules, and is presented to activated helper T cells. B cells are activated to plasma cells by helper T cells, and produce IgM and IgG through affinity maturation, class switching, and discrimination by FDC. Naive killer T cells are activated through cross presentation to MHC class Ⅰ molecules.

The Fc region of IgG binds to the Fc receptor on the surface of immune cells (antigen binds to the Fab region of the antibody), and the immune cells violently eat the antigen. That is, they fight against antigens through opsonization and neutralization. Opsonization is the action that the Fc receptor of phagocytic cells binds to the FC region of IgG and the phagocytic cells can efficiently eat the antigen, and this is called the opsonization effect of antibodies. Neutralization is the ability of antibodies to bind to toxins or viruses to reduce toxicity. Activated killer cells open holes in infected cells and inject enzymes to cause apoptosis, and induce apoptosis by pushing the apoptosis switch. Furthermore, innate immune cells and natural killer cells destroy infected cells in the same way as killer T cells.

Factors that may exacerbate infection immunity

Macrophage: It occupies 5% of leucocytes, and are derived from monocytes. Monocytes differentiate from hematopoietic stem cells, mature in the bone marrow, enter the bloodstream, stay in the bloodstream for two days, then enter tissues and become macrophages.

Neutrophil: Account for 45-75% of leucocytes and have strong phagocytic ability along with macrophage.

Lymphocytes: 2000-2300 cells/μliter or more is said to be sufficient for immunity.

B cells: 20-40% of lymphocytes are B cells.

T cells: Progenitor cells produced in the bone marrow differentiate in the thymus. They present in the thymus. It accounts for 60-80% of lymphocytes. T cells comprise CD4-positive T cells (300-1300/μL in number) and CD8 positive (suppressive) T cells (100-900/μL).

Mutations and deletions of TLR, RLR, CLR, NLR, cGAS, etc. in pattern recognition cells.

Cytokines, chemokines.

MyD88: A gateway molecule for immune system signaling in phagocytic cells, which culminates in NFκB through various pathways. It is a signaling substance essential for Interleukin 1 and the TLR signaling pathway, and is a type of intracellular adapter protein that promotes the activation of signaling molecules. Lack of MYD88 makes it vulnerable to infection. Adaptor protein is a kind of protein involved in signal transduction, and mediates association between receptor and signal transduction molecule although it does not have enzymatic activity.

Co-stimulatory factor CD28 in naive cells.

Besides that: MHC class II molecule, Co-stimulatory factor CD80/86 of dendritic cells.

These factors mentioned above do not always work perfectly either quantitatively or qualitatively. The process by which viruses invade cells is often described, and the following two routes are well known.

1. ACE2 receptor pathway

For organs that have ACE2 receptors (ACE1 is related to hypertension), spikes of the new coronavirus enter cells from the ACE2 receptors (generally, the new coronavirus is infected through this route).

2. FC receptor pathway

For some reason, most cases of ADE occurring via Fc receptors in immune cells occur via this route. In other words, the Fcγ receptor of macrophages and the Fc region of immunoglobulin IgG (incompletely neutralizing antibody) + antigen (virus) bind to infect macrophages with viruses. The function of the Fc region is called effector function. Since Fcγ receptors have low affinity (weak binding force), opsonization is promoted and activated (phenomenon that antigens are easily taken up by phagocytic cells due to binding of antibodies and complement to antigens. Complement hydrolyzes viruses that have taken up into macrophage by phagocytosis).

§3 Treatment for covid 19

There are still no antiviral drugs or vaccines that are as accurate as drug therapy for bacteria. Let's start with antiviral drugs. There is no silver bullet that shows significant efficacy. In other words, there is no choice but to treat with drug repositioning. In other words, it is a last resort to discover new medicinal effects from existing drugs and connect them to practical use as novel coronavirus therapeutics.

1. Remdesivir (Veklury): An antiviral drug originally used to treat Ebola hemorrhagic fever. For moderately ill patients. Administer within 7 days of onset. Although it is a typical drug that exhibits antiviral effects, no significant effect on mortality was observed in the WHO SOLIDARITY trial.

2. Molnupiravir (Lagevrio): A nucleic acid antimetabolite, administered orally within 5 days of onset of symptoms. Patients other than severe cases, within 5 days of onset. It exerts antiviral effects by inhibiting RNA-dependent RNA polymerase enzymes and impeding viral RNA replication.

3. Dexamethasone (for moderate to severe cases) A typical drug for excessive inflammatory reactions.

4. Neutralizing antibody therapy: Administer within 7 days. A mixture of two antibodies (casirivimab and imdevimab), a cocktail of two monoclonal antibodies: casirivimab binds to the spike protein's receptor binding site in a non-competitive manner, and imdevimab binds to a different site on the spike protein to exert its effect.

5. Sotrovimab (Zebudi): Monoclonal antibody, intravenous administration.

6. Nilmatrevir/ritonavir (Paquirovid): A combination drug of nilmatrevir, a 3CL protease inhibitor, and ritonavir, which enhances its effect, used together within 5 days of onset of symptoms. Only for seriously ill patients. There are 40 drugs that are prohibited from being used together. Dosage must be adjusted for patients with decreased renal function.

7. Ensitrelvir (Zocova): 3CL protease inhibitor, oral medication.

8. Tocilizumab (Actemra): Anti-IL-6 receptor antibody (used for rheumatoid arthritis, Takayasu arteritis).

9. Futhan (nafamostat): It prevents the fusion of the outer membrane of the virus with the cells. It has been used as a treatment for acute pancreatitis.

10. Favipiravir (Avigan): Development has been discontinued.

Most of the above medications are not suitable for asymptomatic patients or those with mild symptoms.

Concerning increase in severity of new coronavirus infection, people with underlying diseases, as mentioned below, are more likely to develop severe symptoms: Elderly with underlying diseases, obesity, cardiovascular disease, asthma, DM, chronic renal failure, chronic liver disease, immunosuppressive conditions (malignant disease, HIV [CD4 < 200/μL]).

Respiratory therapy is an important part of treatment, and in severe cases it can affect life prognosis. Nasal cannula or mask O_2 administration to maintain $SpO_2 > 93$ as the severity increases, and if unable to maintain $SpO_2 > 93$, mask with reservoir 10-15 L/min or nasal high flow (30L-40L/min) (to prevent aerosol generation, negative pressure private room is recommended). Use intubated ventilators for ARDS, muscle relaxants for excessive spontaneous breathing efforts, and closed endotracheal suctioning. L-type (mild) is deeply sedated with PEEP 8-10 cmH_2O. For type H (severe), PEEP 10-14 cmH_2O and prone position ventilation were used to treat ARDS. ECMO, blood purification therapy (absorption and removal of inflammatory cytokines in preparation for progression of multiple organ failure).

Seven days after the onset those with mild symptoms were further relieved. Those with severe symptoms who had only normal cold symptoms until 7 days after onset, and their respiratory function worsened after 7 days were hospitalized, and some were admitted to the ICU.

Regarding the coronavirus vaccine, Professor Jennifer Doudna of the University of California at Berkeley and Dr. Emmanuel Charpentier of EU Max Planck Institute were awarded the Nobel Prize in Chemistry for genome editing technology in 2020. Professor Katalin Kariko and Professor Drew Weissman of the University of Pennsylvania contributed to the creation of the new coronavirus vaccine and are awarded the Nobel Prize in Physiology or Medicine for this in 2023. The Pfizer and Moderna vaccines created based on their research is called mRNA vaccines. They decode the gene sequence that makes the spike protein of the new coronavirus and create mRNA that will serve as the blueprint for making spike protein in human cells. The generated mRNA is encapsulated in lipid nanoparticles and injected into the muscle. The virus's spike protein is produced in muscle cells and dendritic cells according to the mRNA blueprint and stimulates the human immune system. As a result, cells have the same spike protein as the new coronavirus. In other words, a vaccine containing mRNA that has the blueprint for only the protruding part (spike protein) of the new coronavirus is injected into the muscle, and amino acids are synthesized based on the blueprint of the mRNA taken into cells to create the spike protein. The body's immune system recognizes this spike protein and mounts an immune response such as producing antibodies against it.

Concerning side effects of corona vaccine, anaphylaxis is rare but usually occurs in women. MRNA is encapsulated in a lipid + nanomolecule (LNP). Side effect is due to the use of polyethylene glycol PEG to preserve the water solubility of the LNP lipid bilayer. In the case of women, it is related to the fact that they had previously been sensitized by cosmetics. It is also used as an additive in medicines and foods.

§4 Immune memory

Immunological memory is an immune mechanism that recognizes the encountered antigens and initiates subsequent immune responses. Both B and T cells include memory B cells, memory killer T cells, and memory helper T cells. First, these naive B cells, naive killer T cells, and naive helper T cells (cells that have not yet encountered antigen are called naive cells) are activated by antigen stimulation and proliferate, and are called effector cells. Some of them become memory cells. These memory cells continue to live, and when antigens invade again, they can be activated and produce a rapid response. Thus, antibody production and effector T cell activity are rapidly increased.

Three types of memory B cells

① High-affinity IgG-type memory B cells

High-affinity IgG-type memory B cells have undergone class switching and high-affinity maturation. It takes 2 to 3 weeks for antibody production to reach its peak in the first infection, but when it becomes memory B cells after the initial infection, these memory B cells can produce a large amount of antibody in about 4 days. They differentiate into antibody-producing cells called plasma cells that produce antibodies that can strongly bind to antigens re-invading, which are the main force of memory B cells. Some become B cells instead of becoming plasma cells. The reason why plasma cells can quickly produce large amounts of antibodies is that the number of memory B cells increases after the first stimulation, and the differentiation is progressing. Memory B cells are much closer to plasma cells than naive B cells. However, their proliferative capacity is inferior to that of naive B cells. However, since the number is increasing, the time to reach the peak of antibody production is short and the amount of antibody is large. Moreover, it is thought that there may be memory helper T cells near memory B cells. Furthermore, among the high-affinity IgG-type plasma cells, those that migrate to the bone marrow have a significantly longer lifespan. These are called long-lived plasma cells.

② Low-affinity IgG-type memory B cells

They have undergone class switching but have not undergone affinity maturation.

③ Low-affinity IgM-type memory B cells

They have not undergone class switching or affinity maturation.

For these three types of memory B cells (Akira S, Kurosaki T: New introduction to immunity. Kodansha Tokyo, 2014); ① are the main force of memory B cells and differentiate into plasma cells that produce antibodies that can strongly bind when antigens re-invade. ② correspond to antigen mutation. For example, in the case of influenza, when re-infected the following year, the incidence of infection with a newly mutated virus, unlike the previous virus, is very high. However, the antibodies that already existed before infection have weak binding to newly mutated antigens. Nevertheless, these low-affinity IgG-type memory B cells undergo affinity maturation after infection with the mutated influenza virus, and they are likely to produce antibody which strongly bind to mutated antigens. ③ do not differentiate into plasma cells and serve as a supply source to prevent depletion of IgG-type memory B cells.

Memory B cells are of plasma cell origin and its peak in antibody production is 2 weeks after infection. Memory T cells stay in the body for years.

Furthermore, follicular dendritic cells (FDC) may play an important role in immunological memory (the surface molecule CR2, which is a complement receptor, plays a role).

Speaking of memory T cells, there are two types of helper T cells and killer T cells: effector memory T cells and central memory T cells. There are many effector memory T cells in the periphery (mucosal organs such as the lungs, trachea, and intestines), and they can quickly exhibit effector functions when antigens enter again, but their proliferation ability is poor and their lifespans are short.

Central memory T cells are abundant in lymph nodes. Central memory T cells cannot exert effector functions immediately, but they have a high proliferative capacity. It has a long lifespan and prepares for the next infection.

After the primary immune response ends, effector cells are eliminated, but antibodies, memory T cells, and memory B cells remain. Memory T cells stay in the body for years. It can last for decades in the body. Chickenpox, measles, etc. last a lifetime, and this is called lifelong immunity. It is well known that dengue fever and the like often cause antibody-dependent enhancement of infection at the next infection. Even for diseases that are supposed to cause lifelong immunity, neutralizing antibodies may actually become negative unless subclinical infections are repeated. Less than 30 years for mumps and less than 6 months for influenza is the limit of immunity effectiveness.

§5 Antibody-dependent enhancement (ADE)

This is a well-known phenomenon that has gained attention due to the increase in severity of the disease when reinfected with dengue fever. If you are infected with dengue fever Type Ⅰ, you will develop neutralizing antibodies that will prevent reinfection for the rest of your life (the same phenomenon occurs with measles and rubella). However, evidence shows that if you contract another type of dengue fever, such as Type II, the Type II virus may bind to the Type I antibody, forming an immune complex which may not neutralize the virus and could exacerbate the infection. The phenomenon has been known to occur. In addition to the novel coronavirus, other enveloped RNA viruses include members of the Flaviviridae family, which have frequently caused ADE, and there is concern that the novel virus may also cause it. In other words, since the new coronavirus is closely related to the Flaviviridae family that has caused ADE, there are concerns that it will cause ADE in the same way.

ADE is caused by endocytosis via FC receptors of Fc receptor-bearing cells, including immune cells. First, viruses bound to the Fc region of IgG bind to FcγR, in short, the FcγR (Fcγ receptor) pathway. This receptor is on the surface of immune cells. The low affinity binding to this receptor promotes opsonization and is activated. Opsonization is a phenomenon in which an antibody or complement binds to an antigen, making it easier for the antigen to be taken up by phagocytic cells. Macrophage takes this complex into the cell by endocytosis. Complement should normally hydrolyze the ingested virus.

In addition, if I say:

1. Coronaviruses enter cells: either via the ACE II receptor or via the Fc receptor (mostly the former). The ADE phenomenon is mediated only by the latter (IgG→Fcγ receptor). In other words, when ADE occurs, the infection is via the FCγRII receptor of macrophages. Since this receptor has low affinity and weak avidity, opsonization is promoted and activated. Alternatively, spike proteins may bind and enter via the complement pathway (which is still not very well understood).
2. The virus becomes an antigen and forms a complex with an incompletely neutralizing antibody that was produced in the past in IgG (there is no neutralizing power, but there is adsorption power to Fc receptors), resulting in endocytosis (phagocytosis). ADE is a phenomenon in which this complex enters immune cells through the Fc receptor pathway and enhances replication within the cells. Then, it enhances the replication ability in the cell and enhances the infection. A new antigen (virus) binds to an existing incompletely neutralizing antibody that has no neutralizing ability but has adsorptive power, forms a complex, and enters immune cells such as macrophages. The same thing can happen with vaccination. ADE can occur from either primary or secondary viral infection or post-vaccination.
3. Due to cross-reactivity between previous coronavirus infection and this new coronavirus, incomplete pre-existing IgG antibodies (low neutralizing ability) may exacerbate ADE. ADE tends to have a long latency period (6.6% with a latency period of 14 days or longer) because it is often cross-reactive.
4. High blood IgG levels starting from the very early stage of infection call attention to a phenomenon of cross-reactivity of residual incomplete antibodies due to the presence of memory of previous infection.
5. There are no known clinical findings, immunological assays, or biomarkers that distinguish severe viral infection from ADE. Even in vitro, it is impossible to predict the risk of ADE in disease. Because the mechanisms of ADE and normal immune reactions are almost the same.
6. In order to prevent ADE, it is necessary to create a powerful vaccine, not a half-baked vaccine with a low antibody titer. Ingenuity of adjuvants and intramuscular injection for adjuvant is required. There are two types of antibodies: neutralizing antibodies (which bind to toxins) and infectious antibodies (antibodies produced by the body as a result of infection that do not necessarily neutralize). Antibodies are a mixture of neutralizing antibodies and infection-enhancing antibodies, so when making a vaccine, it is necessary to mutate them to weaken the infection-enhancing antibodies.
7. The incomplete antibody and the virus made in the past combine and this complex is taken up by macrophage by endocytosis (phagocytosis).

If the basic reproduction number is 2 to 3, herd immunity means that 60% of the population has immunity. As of January 2021, 63 vaccines were in clinical trials. Covid 19 mutates quickly and the period in which vaccines are effective has a very short. A third of patients who recovered from covid 19 have only small amount of antibodies. Antibodies may not play such a large role in the immune system, as it is likely that innate immunity alone has been expected to cure the disease. That's why it's so hard to get herd immunity.

In the first place, the new coronavirus infection in Japan is;

1. Attenuated bacteria unlike those in Europe and the United States. Since most Japanese already have antibodies and cellular immunity, many patients do not develop symptoms. The designated infectious disease was changed from Category 2 to Category 5 (May 2023).
2. Covid 19 has S, K and G types. Type S entered Japan first, followed by type K, which then spread throughout Japan, causing a phenomenon called viral interference, which suppressed the epidemic of influenza. Mortality

has declined as the K strain has spread and strengthened immunity, resulting in acquirement of considerable herd immunity to covid 19.

3. Covid 19 has 80% homology with the SARS virus and 50% with the cold coronavirus, and the current situation in Japan is that the immune memory of past cold coronaviruses functions as cross-immunity against covid 19.

§6 Immune mechanism in covid 19

Humoral immunity is the main component of viral infection at first, but cellular immunity becomes important thereafter. Among cell-mediated immunity, killer T cells (cytotoxic T cells, CTL) are important. CTLs have CD8 molecules on the surface of naive killer T cells. Dendritic cells with MHC class Ⅰ molecules bound to degraded antigen bind to killer T cells. The dendritic cells are in a state in which the antigen bound to the class 1 molecule and the antigen + class II molecule are bound. Helper T cells release cytokines to killer T cells, or dendritic cells release a large amount of cytokines to killer T cells, and naive killer T cells are activated.

First, the incompletely neutralizing antibody acquired by the patient does not have neutralizing power, but it has the ability to adsorb to Fc receptors. The incompletely neutralizing antibody make a complex, binding to an antigen (virus) invading anew. ADE is a phenomenon that forms the complex, which enters cells via the Fc receptor pathway, and enhances the ability to replicate within cells.

A new antigen (virus) binds to an already existing incomplete neutralizing antibody that has no neutralizing ability but has adsorptive power, forms a complex, and enters immune cells such as macrophages. This can also occur with vaccines.

"Original antigen sin" is a reaction to a known antigen (the patient was infected this time, but he had a history of similar infection in the past, and the current antigen reacted to immunity to the previous antigen). This is because there is a memory of cross-reactivity when IgG appears early in infection and shows high levels. It's just boosting antibodies against old antigens, not recognizing new antigens, causing ADE. Early high levels of IgG due to cross-reactivity between previous coronavirus infection and the current novel coronavirus may have already exacerbated ADE. Finally, T cells that expose Fas molecules to the surface bind to Fas ligands from other cells, and the T cells undergo apoptosis and become necrotic.

When ADE occurs, the viruses bind to spike protein and enter through the FCγRII receptor or through the complement pathway (the complement pathway is still not very clearly understood). Because cross-reactivity is common, the incubation period tends to be long (6.6% had an incubation period of 14 days or longer).

Concerning antibodies, neutralizing antibodies and infection-enhancing antibodies that increase infectivity (Lieu Y, et al: Cell 184:3452, 2021) are produced in combination. Another type of ADE of infection, which occurs through different mechanism described above occurs independently of the Fc receptor and is unrelated to the receptor binding domain (RBD) of the spike protein. Infection-enhancing antibodies can influence after primary or secondary viral infection or after vaccination.

§7 Mutation of the new coronavirus

D614G is the beginning of all the novel coronavirus mutations. This is the first strain that was mutated from the Wuhan strain, that is, the strain that was born by mutation, and is the highly contagious strain D614G, which was the beginning of the global epidemic, and was detected on January 24, 2020. Why are newly emerging mutant strains so highly contagious? This is called the founder effect, and as a result of a relatively small number of individuals (founders) separating from the original population and proliferating in isolation from the original population, a new population (new strain) that is genetically different from the original population are formed that are more contagious than conventional strains.

What is the cause of the mutation? 1. Mutation due to miscopy during viral replication. 2. Antibodies are produced by vaccination, and when the virus is neutralized, the virus mutates in an attempt to avoid neutralization (escape from the neutralizing antibody) (this is called immune escape, and the effect of the vaccine is reduced because it escapes the antibody). 3. The same mutation is emerging on three different continents. That is, although three different mutations (N501Y, E484K, K417) appeared independently in different lineages on three different continents, the same mutation was associated with the receptor binding domain (RBD) of the S protein. There is a fact that they share the same mutation in the receptor binding region in the spike protein. It is thought that this is not a coincidence, but the result of inevitable "convergent evolution." The convergent evolution refers to a phenomenon in which living body of different lineages acquire similar traits even if they are from different lineages when their ecological environments are similar.

Since then, through various mutations, various phenomena have come to be seen in this process. That is, it spreads 50-70% faster. Children are more likely to become infected. Infectivity is 1.7 times higher than before. It reduces the production of neutralizing antibodies by a tenth. The induced antibodies in current vaccines bind to subspecies instead of the original strain and do not neutralize the original strain. It has been said that young people are susceptible to infection, fear of reinfection, easy transmission of infection, and high resistance to vaccines.

Currently, the number of new coronaviruses is gradually decreasing, but the number of mutant strains is increasing. For details, there are many mutations in the spike protein, mutation to a virus with the ability to escape from neutralizing antibodies (having the ability to escape from neutralizing antibodies), concerns about ADE, concerns about reinfection, and becoming endemic, increased mortality, increased juvenile population among thc patients, mutations not found in PCR tests. Mutant strains affect neutralization by polyclonal and monoclonal antibodies. Mutant strains cause conformational change of spike protein (change in three-dimensional structure of protein) and polarization of amino acids.

The immune evasion mechanism of the virus uses properly up-regulation and down-regulation of the immune response ability.

Corona's innate immune evasion is done by the following three; 1. Evasion from receptor recognition. 2. Inhibits interferon transcription. 3. Inhibits type I interferon signal transduction.

Why does the new coronavirus mutant strain spreads so quickly? It is widely believed that the change in conformation due to mutation strengthens the binding force, which in turn enhances the infectivity.

There are three possible causes of reinfection; 1. The second dose of viral infection is higher than the first. 2. Caused by a more virulent mutant strain. 3. ADE. The time between primary infection and reinfection is short (although one should usually be immune for 5 months). It is doubtful whether mechanisms such as memory B lymphocytes and memory T lymphocytes are at work.

Finally, it can be said that the current infection status of covid 19 has generally calmed down. 40-50% of all infected people are asymptomatic, and the asymptomatic infected people's immunity declines faster and drops sharply in 2-3 months. In younger children symptoms are milder and overall is asymptomatic. It is believed that covid 19 may have caused a vaccine-escape mutation. Booster shots provide effective protection against mutant strains (Pfizer's opinion). Current PCR tests are not sufficient to detect mutant strains. The covid 19 killed 70,000 people in Japan and 7 million people worldwide so far.

Index (words on the pages of the table of contents are omitted from the following indexes)

Brief histories of ourselves

Dr. Masaharu Sato is currently the director of Takarazuka Rehabilitation Hospital. He graduated from Shinshu University Medical School in 1974. He is originally a neurosurgeon and began his clinical experience at Department of Neurosurgery Osaka University, where he obtained his board certification in neurosurgery. After that, he conducted experimental research on cerebral circulation and metabolism at Max-Planck Institut für Hirnforschung (Prof. WD. Heiss) in Cologne, West Germany for 2 years. He received Medical Doctor Thesis (Osaka University Medical School) (Prof. T . Hayakawa) in 1985. Afterwards, clinical work on head injury and stroke was conducted at Department of Emergency Medicine Kawasaki Medical University (Prof. A. Kohama, Prof. C. Fujii) for 4 years. In addition, he was engaged in clinical work on brain tumors, stroke, pediatric neurosurgery, and experimental research on cerebral circulation and metabolism at Department of Neurosurgery Kinki University (Prof. M. Ioku) for 4.5 years. Further, clinical work on brain tumor and aneurysm surgery has been conducted at Toyonaka Municipal Hospital Stroke Center as chairman. He has specialist's qualifications from Japanese Society of Neurosurgery, Society of Stroke, Society of Emergency Medicine (former), Society of Dementia, and Society of Rehabilitation. He is also an active member of International Congress of CBF and Metabolism. Currently, as a culmination of these basic to clinical experiences, he is focusing on the molecular biological change in the convalescent stage.

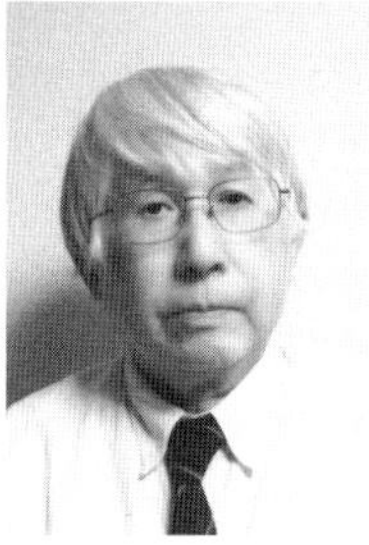

Masaharu Sato

Dr. Junji Taguchi is currently the chief director of Takarazuka Rehabilitation Hospital. He graduated from Ehime University Medical School in 1982. He is also originally a neurosurgeon and began his clinical experience at Department of Neurosurgery Osaka University, where he obtained his board certification in neurosurgery and qualification of specialist from Society of Stroke. He also conducted experimental research on cerebral circulation and metabolism at Max-Planck Institut für neurologische Forschung (Prof. WD. Heiss) in Cologne, West Germany for 2 years. Further, he received Medical Doctor Thesis (Osaka University Medical School) (Prof. T. Hayakawa). After a clinical experience on neurosurgery he was designated a chief director of Takarazuka Rehabilitation Hospital. His clinical research interests include neuroplasticity in stroke at the convalescent stage.

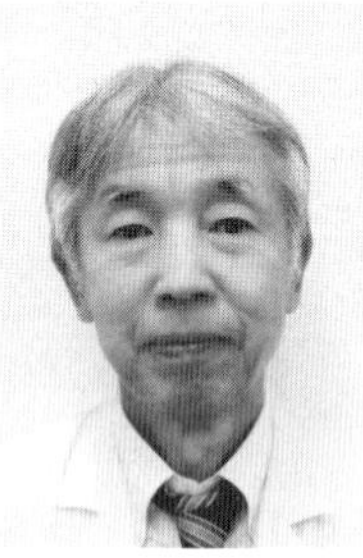

Junji Taguchi

Pathophysiological Basis of Treatment in Convalescent Rehabilitation

2024年10月15日　初版第１刷発行

Author　Masaharu Sato
Editor　Junji Taguchi
発行者　瓜谷 綱延
発行所　株式会社文芸社
〒160-0022 東京都新宿区新宿1－10－1
電話 03-5369-3060（代表）
03-5369-2299（販売）

印刷所　TOPPANクロレ株式会社

ISBN978-4-286-25195-0